I'M GOING TO RUN UNTIL I'M DONE

I'M GOING TO RUN UNTIL I'M DONE

Contending with Cancer
Contending for the Faith

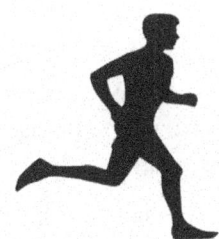

DEANA DICKERSON

I'M GOING TO RUN UNTIL I'M DONE
Copyright © 2022 by Deana Dickerson

All rights reserved. No part of this book may be reproduced in any form or by any electronic or mechanical means, including information storage and retrieval systems, without written permission from the author, except for the use of brief quotations in a book review.

Cover and Interior Design: Living Lights Media, Jason Sisam

Published by Salmon Prairie Press

Scripture quotations are from The ESV® Bible (The Holy Bible, English Standard Version®), copyright © 2001 by Crossway, a publishing ministry of Good News Publishers. Used by permission.

Scripture quotations marked (NIV) are taken from the Holy Bible, New International Version®, NIV®. Copyright © 1973, 1978, 1984, 2011 by Biblica, Inc.™ Used by permission of Zondervan. All rights reserved worldwide. www.zondervan.com The "NIV" and "New International Version" are trademarks registered in the United States Patent and Trademark Office by Biblica, Inc.™

Scriptures marked KJV are taken from the KING JAMES VERSION (KJV): KING JAMES VERSION, public domain/Scripture taken from the New King James Version®. Copyright © 1982 by Thomas Nelson. Used by permission. All rights reserved.

Scriptures marked HCSB are taken from the HOLMAN CHRISTIAN STANDARD BIBLE (HCSB): Scripture taken from the HOLMAN CHRISTIAN STANDARD BIBLE, copyright© 1999, 2000, 2002, 2003 by Holman Bible Publishers, Nashville Tennessee. All rights reserved.

Scriptures marked NLT are taken from the HOLY BIBLE, NEW LIVING TRANSLATION (NLT): Scriptures taken from the HOLY BIBLE, NEW LIVING TRANSLATION, Copyright© 1996, 2004, 2007 by Tyndale House Foundation. Used by permission of Tyndale House Publishers, Inc., Carol Stream, Illinois 60188. All rights reserved. Used by permission.

Scripture quotations taken from the (NASB®) New American Standard Bible®,

Copyright © 1960, 1971, 1977, 1995, 2020 by The Lockman Foundation. Used by permission. All rights reserved.

Scripture taken from the Modern English Version. Copyright © 2014 by Military Bible Association. Used by permission. All rights reserved.

Scripture quotations marked JUB (or JBS) are taken from the Jubilee Bible (or Biblia del Jubileo), copyright © 2000, 2001, 2010, 2013 by Life Sentence Publishing, Inc. Used by permission of Life Sentence Publishing, Inc., Abbotsford, Wisconsin. All rights reserved.

Any emphasis in Scripture quotations are the author's.

"God Leads Us Along" by G. A. Young is in the public domain

ISBN: 979-8-218-06623-9 *(Print Edition)*

Printed in the United States of America

10 9 8 7 6 5 4 3 2 1

DISCLAIMER

This memoir records the author's recollection of actual experiences with the aid of journal notes, running logs, calendar notations, and medical records. Recreated conversations reflect the essence of those interactions.

CONTENTS

CHAPTER 1	1
HITTING THE WALL	
Waiting | *October 12, 2007*	1
Just Words	4
Not on our Radar	5
Home	7
Regroup	10
Pleadings	14
Journey | *A Week Later*	15
Recovery	18
Whack-A-Mole | *Two Days Post Surgery*	20
Interjection | *A Week Later*	21
Holy Packets	25
CHAPTER 2	29
FOCUS	
Years Yet | *November 2007*	29
Valley of the Shadow	34
Clarity	36
Hiatus | *December 2007*	38
Seven Times | *Winter 2007*	40
Buoyed | *March 2008*	43
Rerun | *2008-2009*	45
Another | *May 2010*	47
Wholeness | *July 2011*	50
Plans | *October 2011*	54
Photos of Mike	59
CHAPTER 3	63
CHANGES (STILL RUNNING)	
Trip | *March 2012*	63
New | *September 2012*	64
Shift | *October 2012*	66
Adjust | *Winter 2013*	67
March 2013	69

Hope	*Spring 2013*	70
Strategy	*June 2013*	71
More Gear	*Spring 2014*	73
Stepwise	*Summer 2014*	75
Plodding	*November 2014*	76
Getaway	*November 2014*	78
Design	*Summer 2015*	80
Montana Life	*September 2015*	84
Celebration	*January 2016*	86
A Year	*June 2016*	87
Reflection	91
Again	*August 2016*	94
Scene	*September 2016*	99
Months	*May 2017*	102
August 2017	103
Turnaround	*September 24, 2017*	106

CHAPTER 4   109
THE FINISH LINE

Changes	*September 27, 2017*	109
Home	112
Mobility	*October 2017*	114
Holiday Season	*November 2017*	115
Instructions	118
Days	*December 18*	119
Crossing Over	*December 20*	121
Interval	123
Hole-in-my-Heart	125
View	127
Final Chapter	*January 2018*	129
Afterword	131

APPENDIX I   134
FIGHTING SCRIPTURES

APPENDIX II   140
PROMISE SCRIPTURES

About Deana	211

I'M GOING TO RUN UNTIL I'M DONE

1

HITTING THE WALL

WAITING | *OCTOBER 12, 2007*

We had time to waste. After rising early in our fourth-floor hotel room across the street from the Mayo Clinic, my mind went to breakfast. The consummate planner, I tried to structure the day in my mind. My husband and I had traveled one hundred miles from our Minneapolis home to take things leisurely today. Feeling relieved from my usual packed work and travel schedule, I could relax knowing the only thing on my to-do list this day was our visit to Mayo.

Sleepy Mike followed my lead. Usually setting the pace, he remained quiet, barely talking that day. "Let's find a Starbucks," he finally announced. Each day began with Starbucks at home, brewed from freshly ground Sumatra decaf beans.

Of course, we have to find a Starbucks! How could he think of starting his day without that? Mike had a routine, and I knew not to violate this pattern over the thirty-two years we had been married. That is just how our marriage worked. We were both shot-callers; however, I learned when to step aside early on.

We dressed and took the elevator down to the lower floor of our hotel to Starbucks. Then, capping our coffees, we traversed the street to the atrium of the eleven-floor Gonda building. As we entered, sunlight beamed through the enormous ceiling-to-floor windows. We had experienced the beauty and serenity of this space many times before; Mike had been a patient at Mayo for years. Most of those visits were primarily routine checkups. In past years, Mike considered Mayo visits to the Gonda building pleasant outings, with its beautiful artwork and serene atmosphere. But our previous visit left us with questions. This time, as we descended the marble staircase into the Landow Atrium, even the twenty-eight-foot bronze statue with arms stretching to welcome us to this place of healing seemed like a veiled overture to what was about to happen.

As usual, we heard soothing music over the loudspeakers. Like a thin candy glaze covering all those coming here for healing, it varnished the anxiety lodged within Mike. A live-in-the-present person, he loved to sit in this place to soak in its grandeur and tranquility. I wished I was more like that. Always charting the future and best options, I gave myself little time to sit still and enjoy the present.

If we had been at home, Mike usually would run in the morning, taking his usual route down the Luce Line, an old railroad track converted into a thirty-three-mile trail for running, biking, hiking, and cross-country skiing in the winter months. Mike was not a sometimes runner; he ran every day.

Endorphins must have played a considerable role in his chemistry. He gravitated to outdoor activities: golf, camping, hiking, mountain climbing, and of course, running and marathons. Running was a must for Mike, either embedded in his DNA or he felt scared he would die early like his father from a heart attack or his mother from lung cancer. He also prodded me to exercise, walking my usual mile course in the neighborhood. I preferred to work on my to-do list or just sit and read.

When I first met Mike, he was teaching at the University of Iowa. He had received a full-ride golf scholarship to college, and after earning his degree in physical education, he turned to professional golf. I took lessons, and the rest is history. Maybe the attraction was that we were not at all alike. He was a fast-forward guy who came to decisions quickly, whereas I was analytical, taking my time to get an answer. He thrived on stimulation. I renewed with quiet and reflection.

Although Mike was labeled 'the quiet one' by a mutual acquaintance, he could discuss a topic for hours, especially if it bothered him. He would talk about his feelings, a category most guys wouldn't touch.

In the Gonda Atrium, someone started to play the grand piano. We stopped to listen for a moment. Mike was quiet. Then we made our way to the eight-floor clinic for Mike's appointment. Checking in, we settled into color-coordinated upholstered chairs and quietly waited until they called Mike's name. I saw a room full of people also waiting. I briefly wondered what their stories were.

We were at Mayo that day to hear the results of the biopsies taken from the previous visit. Mike's internist scheduled that procedure after detecting something. "This should be nothing to worry about and is usually benign and treatable," the doctor had said.

Finally, we heard Mike's name called. As the nurse guided us down the hall, she queried Mike's full name and birthdate. Confirming his identity, she pointed us into one of the many consultation rooms. "The doctor will be in shortly."

JUST WORDS

This day had begun with the sun beaming into our hotel room. Each time we stayed at this hotel, we remarked how comfortable and serene we felt with its well-appointed lobby and staff looking after our every need. This hotel offered some peace to needy visitors. Most of all, I loved the familiarity of this home-away-from-home.

That peaceful setting sat across the street from where we were now at the clinic. My mind tried to order the events that brought us here today. *Why am I so uneasy? Isn't this appointment going to be routine, like many others at this place?* Up to this point, we had lived at a quiet, steady pace with a few minor bumps. I hoped this was nothing, and we would ride home and pick up where we left off.

The door swung open, and the urologist entered and introduced himself as he shook our hands. He sat down in front of his computer to open Mike's chart. He explained Mayo Clinic takes many more biopsies than other clinics to ensure a complete picture. *That's impressive.* I liked their thoroughness. No stone unturned.

After more explanations of their comprehensive approach, he added, "Mike, we found all the biopsies are malignant. We took eighteen biopsies from all the different lobes, and that is our finding." Then, not to leave us without hope, he added, "But don't worry, I can do surgery as soon as possible if you agree, and if there are no other findings, you will do very well. That is my experience. We have many patients living years after this type of surgery."

I guess that was as much as he could offer at the time. They must do this every day, informing people they have cancer. In just those few words, the moment materialized, taking the stuff of our lives to a place we did not want it to go. A sinkhole, the pronouncement that my husband had cancer!

With this weighty statement, we felt flattened. Like in a cartoon, we had to be scraped off the floor and reconstituted by the doctor. I could not believe what he said about my husband of thirty-two years, the love of my life, and my best friend! Mike was my pillar, my sounding board, my share-it-all soulmate. So unreal, so sudden, this word *malignant* echoed through a tunnel in our ears. It boomeranged in our heads with no way of escape. *I want this so not to be true. How did we get here?* I felt my heart beating fast in my clenched fists.

NOT ON OUR RADAR

Leaning forward in his chair beside the doctor's desk, Mike exclaimed, "I am fit. I run every day, hundreds of miles this last year! I just ran a half-marathon in May and Grandma's Marathon in June! How could this happen?"

I was hard-pressed to understand this incredulous happening as well. I could second that Mike was a healthy guy and was at his fittest at sixty-one years old. His last checkup had been fourteen months earlier. They had checked his blood for the prostate cancer tumor marker(PSA), which was in the normal range. With no symptoms in the intervening time, we did not anticipate what we'd just heard. Eighteen samples and all were positive for prostate cancer.

We were stunned, numb to the rest of the doctor's words. I needed to regroup. *Let me out of this claustrophobic conference room.* Hot all over, I wanted to strip off my outer jacket. I needed to breathe. A rush of adrenalin flooded me. I hoped I would not faint as I had many times in my younger days due to low blood pressure.

The doctor broke our distress. "What questions do you have?"

In my mind, I hammered, *You're the answer-man. You are the top doc here. What questions are we supposed to be asking? Help us out here!*

"Why wouldn't I have symptoms? Wouldn't there have been some clue?" Mike queried.

"Perhaps, not in all cases."

"But I don't understand how this happened so fast. My checkup last year, my PSA was okay."

"PSA is the prostate serum antigen found in normal as well as malignant cells of the prostate gland. The actual number of the PSA marker can be just that. It is not the absolute number we consider. What is significant is the doubling of that PSA number, even if the number is low. Your PSA went from 1 to 4 in a little over a year. I recommend we do surgery as soon as possible. If there is no cancer outside the prostate gland, you will do excellent." Mike nodded agreement to surgery.

"Let's get you set up the surgery scheduler." The doctor continued. "Our front desk will arrange for that. I will see you soon."

This urologist would be Mike's surgeon. He shook our

hands and left the room. The nurse ushered us back to the large, airy waiting room front desk, where I could breathe again. With the cool air of the waiting room flooding over me, we waited for further instructions.

"Someone will contact you as soon as the surgery schedule is confirmed," the receptionist said.

We both needed to escape this place as fast as possible.

"I just don't understand," Mike uttered as we left for the elevator. He moved fast as I tried to catch up.

"Mike, wait!" I ran to catch up to him. Searching for words to combat this devastating news, I had none. *How did this happen to our tidy life?*

On the elevator, I started to feel the intense heaviness of the moment—like a dusty black velvet stage curtain lowering over our lives with an audience stunned at the ending. No one clapped.

HOME

We got on the elevator and rode down in silence. "Lobby Level," the pleasant elevator voice announced at our arrival on the main floor. With the words we had just heard, I felt leveled. Thoughts whirling out of control, my mind tried to get some order. I could not curb the rush of calamitous consequences I imagined could happen.

We sat in our hotel café, trying to understand what had just transpired. Neither of us was hungry. My poor Mikey. His usual sunny outlook had disappeared. *What can I say to ease the pain of this terrible news?* My own raw heart hemorrhaged. How often had I told family and friends when they were going through a challenging time—the shortest prayer is just crying the name 'Jesus.' That thought never came to me.

I came from a line of courageous women. They unflappably rose to meet the challenges before them. I knew my mother must have been overwhelmed with my father's sudden passing, leaving her with four young children. I saw her faint at the funeral visitation in our home, where they carried her out on a stretcher. Later, I saw her rise to manage farms and businesses. I also knew she'd stood stalwart in the hospital during the weeks she watched my brother die, her firstborn and only son. But I did not feel fearless at this moment.

Inside, I was limp, and my heart agonized. My usual armadillo outer façade was cracking. The three words that people dread hearing, "You have cancer," pierced our idyllic life. The doctor did not say those exact words, but he might as well have. I felt the stab. Paralyzed for words, I searched for anything to say that would be of comfort. This news felt like a dark storm cloud gathering over us. I sensed we were about to get drenched.

As we left town, Mike drove with tears spilling down his face. He exclaimed he could not believe he had cancer after working to be healthy. He began reviewing all the great pains he'd taken, never to hear those words. Exercising since his twenties, his plan, *our* plan, was to grow old together. I added how heart-healthy his diet was and how careful we were. We wouldn't even eat pizza, Mike's favorite food, more than once a month.

"I tried so hard to stay so healthy, and now this?"

"You did everything right." But inside, I, too, questioned what might have caused this. But, more than that, I realized this situation was not in our control.

We arrived home. Our peaceful cul-de-sac looked the same, but we were not the same. Our façade brick home, with its arched entry and perfectly manicured lawn, welcomed us back. We entered our west-facing kitchen-family-room area and deposited our overnight bags. This bright space offered a cheery hello, even though we did not reciprocate.

A natural reaction should be for us to get on our knees and pray. But we didn't go there. The shocking news took our focus completely off God. Instead, my brain focused on the flashing neon light blinking, 'CANCER!' We should have been imploring the Lord in our distress. This new scenario silenced us.

This slap in the face launched a long, uninvited detour into a chapter we would not choose. Yet, something told me this unwanted foreigner named "Cancer" was settling in and making itself comfortable. In our minds, this new presence confronted us at every turn, yelling, "I am here for the long haul. Make room."

We settled into our talking room, the sun porch, a place where Mike always had his coffee and read his Bible in the mornings. Windows on all sides, this sanctuary became our place for peace, a space beckoning us more than any other room in the house. No TV or electronics, just a couple of chairs, a couch and coffee table, and expansive views of the surrounding landscape and marsh.

I positioned myself in a chair next to him. "Two sets of ears are always better than one," I began. Most of the way home, I had been paralyzed for words to say—paralyzed by scenarios that terrified me. Deluged with fear, I tried to stay on a superficial level, not for him but me, for I was near tears.

"Sometimes, we may miss something the other heard." We

started a rehash of everything the doctor had said, hoping for some balm to cover the raw wound we both felt.

"I don't understand it," Mike agonized. "I just had a checkup, not more than a year ago! They said everything was okay." I heard his pleading voice as tears rolled down his cheeks again.

"I know," tears spilled out as I jumped up and put both arms around him.

"I had no symptoms?"

"I know. Do you remember anything at all that would have been a clue?"

"Not a thing. I just ran a half-marathon and a full marathon this summer! You'd think something would show up. And I am at my best weight since high school."

"If anyone lives a clean life, you do."

"Lot of good that does for me now."

"You know," I remembered, "the doctor said, if they get it all, you'll do excellent," hoping to lift his spirits and mine. I desperately needed to talk with God now. So my prayer became for God to contain it, confine it, and fence it in. But would He?

REGROUP

The following day, I arose early and made coffee. As I did, I heard a noise from upstairs that indicated Mike was up. I waited for him on our sun porch. The sunlight streamed through the tilted blinds, brightening the whitewashed pine paneling lining the walls and cathedral ceiling. It was our little chapel. As he entered the kitchen, his mood was evident. He poured his coffee, then took his place on the porch couch and just sat there. Usually, he would pick up his Bible and read a chapter.

From the early years of our marriage, I knew that he was not as familiar with all the verses in the Old Testament that charged us to be strong and fear not. I learned many of these verses from attending years of Sunday School. Like Joshua, who exhorted the children of Israel to be strong and not afraid when they approached the enemy as they went in to conquer the promised land, we were now facing a new enemy we could not see.

I saw in my mother how trust in God was a way of life. I learned bedtime prayers early, attended church and Sunday School without fail each week, and went to a Christian camp for a week each summer. My mother read all those Bible stories to our family, and I memorized many short Bible verses. Scripture and songs became an integral part of my life throughout my childhood. My mother taught us to ask God to lead and direct every area of our lives and talk with Him even about the small details. When I was eleven, I decided to follow Jesus as Lord of my life. I remember that evening evangelistic service when the Lord stirred my heart. There was no dramatic conversion on that November evening in my youth, only a touched heart.

Mike had a different story. Unlike me, he didn't attend Sunday School or church in his youth. He came from a secular home and had no actual knowledge of the Bible during his younger days. Then, in his mid-twenties, his life went downhill. When I first met him, I wondered how he had gained such wisdom so early in life. Coming off divorce with barely more than the clothes on his back, his winning smile and sunny disposition belied prior wounds. After all that heartache, I learned that he had become a believer just six months before I met him. And I also learned of a seasoned mentor, his father's best friend, who took him under his wings after Mike's father's death. When Mike's life seemed to be falling apart, he had nothing else but to trust God. He recalls walking down a street with little money in his pocket for his next meal and crying out, "God, I need help."

From that day forward, he turned his life over to God. He changed and became thirsty for the Word of God. After we were married, he became like a kid in a candy store reading Bible stories about Abraham, Moses, and David. He had never heard of these accounts. "Think of it," he exclaimed, "Abraham, hearing from God to leave his country and move to an unknown land, just pick up and go!" I loved our long conversations following Mike's reading of the Word about these faith heroes. These characters of old persevered through tough times, yet the hand of God was on them.

I kept a recipe file of handwritten Scripture verses over the years. Many of these cards were now dog-eared from much use over my long career in the cardiovascular field. I'd place a card in my suit pocket in the morning before I left for work. When I reached my hand in my pocket, that card reminded me that God walked with me through whatever I faced that day. Through these verses, I relied on the Lord to keep me strong during demanding work situations.

Earlier that morning, I chose the card with the verse from Joshua 1:9, where Joshua appeals to the children of Israel. *"Be strong and courageous. Do not be afraid; do not be discouraged; for the Lord, your God will be with you wherever you go"* (Joshua 1:9 NIV). Placing it so Mike would see it when he sat down for his coffee, I realized I needed this verse just as much as he did.

Mike scanned the little card and then quickly put it aside. We both needed spiritual reinforcement. We needed undergirding to give us hope. Yet, I began to question if God had abandoned us. It's that feeling of being left hanging out in the whipping wind. We both had experienced abandonment in earlier marriages, so we knew it well.

I remember how alone I felt when my marriage abruptly ended without warning after five months. I never saw it coming—so many questions. I struggled to face my new, sudden reality. In graduate school at that time, I entered a long, low period of barely existing. I could barely move forward. Mike's story was different. His first wife disappeared with their young child without explanation. For decades, he wrestled with this stripping of value. The years of hurt, the empty hole, left life-long marks, and it took decades for him to understand.

"Where is God now?" Mike wanted to know.

"Mikey, He never leaves us. The Bible says that." Yet, I, too, was trying to understand how God could allow this to happen. The world, according to me, was not happening. I had been set up for self-sufficiency and independence early in my life. My father died when I was not quite four years old. Before he died, our morning routine was to have him tie our shoes. One morning, I came downstairs to my father's study den when my mother told my sisters and me, "You will have to learn to tie your own shoes from now on because your father will not be here anymore to do that." I did not comprehend the situation at that young age, but my modus operandi became self-reliance.

But as we sat slogging through this morning-after agony, I knew we had to keep returning to Scripture. God would not abandon us. He knew this episode would happen to us because He knows the end from the beginning. God knew right then how we would get through this. I needed to remember in the Old Testament, He is Jehovah Shammah, the God who is right here, right now.

PLEADINGS

The next day bright daylight broke into our second-floor bedroom windows overlooking the marsh, full of eight-foot cattails already turning brown after a blooming summer. A soft breeze ballooned the sage-colored curtains on either side of the large bedroom window. Mike first saw our house on this cul-de-sac before the construction company put it on the market. Barely able to swing the loan, we jumped for our chance to own such a spot. As we watched neighboring homes erected and sold, they came to life with new families moving onto this peaceful street. Our street, we were told, used to be a meadow full of flowers with pheasants flying around. We awoke in this idyllic setting, our thoughts colliding with our new reality.

After taking our coffees to our sunny porch, I opened the windows to freshen the room. I strategized where our day would go from here. Mike came in and sat down, taking his usual position on the couch. Usually, Mike would be planning his day, beginning with reading the Word, then running. That day, he remained quiet. After his first cup of coffee, he announced, "I'm going running." I saw he wanted to maintain his routine and keep as much normalcy as possible.

"I asked the doctor if I can continue running, and he said by all means."

Mike was not about to give up running, especially when he was in tip-top shape. Those marathon medals displayed in a case showed his heart for staying fit.

"How do you feel?"

"Fine. When do you think Mayo will send the schedule for surgery?"

"I'm hoping they call us today."

Then Mike broke into tears. "Why me? I tried so hard to do everything right, and now this!"

I jumped over to hold him. "Mikey, this is so hard." I tried to console him, but I was crying now, too. "We did not ask for this."

"I know, but I still don't understand."

"You know, the Bible says we will see trouble in this life, but the Lord helps us through it all. We have to hang onto that."

He finished his second cup of coffee and headed to his usual running trail. I knew that I needed to reinforce myself before I could support Mike. I had to lean on God now more than ever. My plan for our life had evaporated. My way provided no answers, only more questions. Overwhelmed by this tsunami we did not see coming, I pleaded with God to help us. I knew He would not let us drown; He would part the waters before us.

I remembered Oswald Chambers wrote in *My Utmost for His Highest*, "The only way God plants His saints is through the whirlwind of His storms."

Yes, we are in the storm now, God. You said, Is anything too hard for Me? Anything? Does anything include cancer?

JOURNEY | *A WEEK LATER*

As I awoke to the morning, I prayed to God for guidance through the days ahead. On this day, we would drive to Mayo Clinic in preparation for Mike's surgery the following day. I wanted God as our source of strength. I wanted His wisdom for the surgeon, a good outcome, and a quick recovery for Mike. Then I left it all in His hands.

As the urologist had explained, they squeezed Mike's case into their surgical schedule as quickly as possible. Earlier I'd emailed both my sisters to pray for God's hand in this surgery and for Mike, his surgeon, and the outcome. Living hours away in Wisconsin and Illinois, they would not be physically present to support us for that day. I had put up a brave front to them, giving them the impression everything was under control. Little did they know how wilted I felt.

I felt our new turn of events poking holes into our ordinary lives, leaving us exposed and depleted. We were leaking with no control whatsoever over this slow drain. More noticeable than that, it wiped out our joy.

Mike gave me cues we were going to carry on as usual. We were not about to give up. "Bring that promise card with us today," Mike requested, referring to a laminated brochure of verses called *God's Promises for Hope and Courage* I had purchased at the church bookstore. I placed it in the car door pocket on my side. As we drove, he said, "Read something to me."

I chose the verse, *"I lift my eyes to the hills. From where does my help come? My help comes from the Lord, who made heaven and earth"* (Psalm 121:1–2, ESV).

"Read another one."

"Even though I walk through the valley of the shadow of death, I will fear no evil, for you are with me; your rod and your staff, they comfort me" (Psalm 23:4, ESV).

Mike's day-before-surgery prep went on all night, with good sleep evading us both. We had instructions to be on one of the upper floors of St. Mary's Hospital at eight a.m. St. Mary's was part of the Mayo campus, just a few blocks from the Gonda building and our hotel. When we arrived at the top-floor surgery suite, it was already a beehive of activity.

I kissed Mike goodbye and asked God to carry him through this surgery and give the urologist wisdom and skill. One of the staff asked me to sit in the surgery waiting room, packed with other patients' family members. Each of us received an identity number so we could watch the screen, which hung high on one side of the room for viewing the progress of our loved one's surgery. I looked for the number assigned to Mike's case. *Pre-surgery prep*, it read. I settled in for what they told me would be two hours maximum. I just sat there with adrenaline to spare.

The morning ticked on with the screen indicating the progression of each patient from surgery to recovery. I saw surgeons enter our waiting room and take family members away to consulting rooms. The screen still indicated Mike was in surgery, so I prayed silently. At eleven o'clock, I remained one of the few family members in the waiting area. The predicted hour-and-a-half-long surgery had turned into an all-morning affair. Finally, at eleven-thirty, Mike's surgeon came out and, in silence, directed me into a tiny consultation room.

We took our seats, and he began to explain. "The surgery took so long because once I removed a lymph node that was cancerous, I removed others for testing."

What? This invader has already traveled outside the prostate gland?

"I am so sorry," he said.

After a long pause, he repeated, "I am so sorry."

Then a third time, he said, "I am so sorry." My mind raced.

What was he trying to tell me? Why wasn't he saying more?

Three times. So sorry. Was he trying to say that he'd done all he could? Was this doctor trying to tell me Mike's life was going to be cut short? How short? Those words closed around me like a net. I could not utter a word.

I recalled when my brother learned he had cancer; he died in three months. I knew now my focus had to be on searching the Word for God's way in our predicament. Mike trusted the Word just like he trusted people. If someone said to him, "I'll call you on Monday," and they did not, they hurt his feelings without knowing it. I realized my charge when I returned home was to scour the Scriptures and my recipe card file for what I called my fighting verses, verses from fighters of the Old Testament who prayed to the Almighty for help, the God who never failed. I wanted the Lord, Himself, to fight for us (Deuteronomy 3:22 NKJV).

RECOVERY

The nurse informed me Mike would take some time to recover from the anesthesia medication. They would move him to a hospital room soon, and if I wanted to get some lunch, now would be a good time. I touched his hand, and he aroused briefly. I wished I could have done more for my poor Mikey at that moment. I knew his pain was under control so that I could leave for lunch, but my mind kept returning to the doctor's words. Their weightiness hovered over me.

I did not want lunch. Instead, I walked around the shops in the basement of the Mayo Clinic. I passed several store windows with lovely merchandise. All the while, my brain tried to make sense of the doctor's words. I replayed those awful words, those "sorry" words, but I could not digest them. Neither could they be eliminated. They remained stuck inside of me. No amount of mental manipulation made them anything but doom.

I began to feel very alone, the uncertainty of everything ahead settling in my heart. I had no control over any of it! I had always thought of myself as a strong person. I felt the opposite now. Others had the impression I had everything together. If they only knew the real me. I am weak, I am frail, I am dust, and I fail.

At this moment, my life's verse came to mind. *"I have set the Lord always before me; because he is at my right hand, I shall not be shaken"* (Psalm 16:8, ESV*).*

I need You, God, now more than ever.

I recalled my mother telling a story about being frightened. She was newly widowed and alone, raising four young children. One night while we were playing on the living room floor, she saw a dark and looming presence outside the front living room window. She turned to her right and realized Jesus, larger than life, stood between the colonnades leading into the dining room with outstretched arms, protecting. I wanted those arms folding around me now, holding me, too.

As I walked around the shops, I vowed never to tell my husband the surgeon's "sorry" words. I had the overwhelming realization my husband might die and soon. Our lives together for three-plus decades have been full up to this point. Yet, in the back of my mind hung a dark overshadowing reality. Cognizant that some latent cancer cells might be in Mike's system floating around, waiting for a place to land, I realized that insidious monster may be silent now but could emerge later.

WHACK-A-MOLE | *TWO DAYS POST SURGERY*

We were in a fight for Mike's life.

I knew, in this life, we will have trouble (John 16:33, NIV). Yet, the Bible tells us the Lord is here for us amid our crisis. He does not want us to fear even though the water seems to cover us (Isaiah 43:1-3 NIV). He wants us to hold on. Perhaps I had been viewing God too casually, keeping Him at arm's length, only grasping for Him when I seriously needed Him. I knew He wanted my entire heart, nothing held back, no idol replacements. My way was not best, not even close. I now wanted to reverse the order and put God first, so I bowed in total submission and surrender.

I could only think of how Jesus meets us in the hard places. I began speaking His words back to Him. I held up His Word before Him, reminding Him of His promises. I began to say His Word *out loud* to Him. Not that He hadn't heard me before, it just helped to reinforce the meaning more clearly to myself.

As I sat by my husband in his hospital room the first morning after surgery, I detected we were in for a struggle. The first-year surgery resident's expression was telling as she and the third-year resident entered Mike's room for morning rounds. She could guess what was ahead for Mike. She had been there during the surgery. She was there as they removed lymph node after lymph node, each sent out for microscopic analysis. She was there when word returned of malignancy in one after another. This young doctor knew the probable course Mike's case would take. No way would I tell Mike what I had gleaned from this morning's doctor rounds. Still under heavy sedation, Mike did not require words now, just my presence. What was I going to tell him when he was ready to talk?

I never allowed the moment to occur. I kept all that to myself. I wanted Mike to have hope for a good recovery.

My sister from Wisconsin came to visit the next day. She brought the support I desperately needed. As we sat by Mike's hospital bed, the nurses came in to let Mike sit up in a chair for the first time. They then left the room. My sister was the first to notice Mike's face washed white. Then he fainted in his chair. My sister bolted to the nurses' desk for help. Getting Mike quickly back in bed, the nurses took his vital signs. Noting his low heart rate, they paged the doctor on the floor. After an ECG and consulting with a cardiologist, they concluded Mike usually had a low heart rate due to his exercise training. Noting the heavy blood loss during surgery, the doctor ordered several units of blood.

Not until evening back at our hotel did I share the doctor's "sorry" statements with my sister and my anxiety that Mike's life would be cut short. It seemed I could fortify myself with Scriptures, but fear kept popping up again, like the old "Whack-a-Mole" carnival games.

I felt helpless to change the course of anything. But with the Lord, I came before Him with tears and pleadings over Mike's life. We had every right to what Jesus accomplished at the Cross and Resurrection—by His stripes, we were healed. I prayed that night for complete healing for Mike.

INTERJECTION | *A WEEK LATER*

After an extended stay in the hospital, we made it home. Mike remained bedridden with his catheter still in place. He was surprised his surgery was so incapacitating. "I cannot believe that just a week ago, I was still running, and now I can barely get out of bed. You are going to have to help me."

"Yes, I have all the instructions. Don't worry." The clinic had equipped me with pages of instructions for administering medications, changing dressings, bathing, disinfecting tubing, and other items. I knew I could handle these tasks. So, taking a week off from work, I became Mike's 24/7 nurse.

I closed the bedroom's blackout window shades so he could sleep as much as possible. Then, as I left our bedroom, I reassured him everything would be okay, "Just rest and recover."

I was off work, so I fervently delved into my new role, knowing I was good at taking charge. Kicking my moccasins and socks off, I sat at the kitchen table and reviewed the instructions again. They did not seem onerous. I felt confident I could handle them all. Then, setting them aside, I welcomed the opportunity to do a bit of neglected housework I had been ignoring. Washing our bedroom comforter became first on the list. Then, after loading the washer with soap, I squashed in the king-sized bedcover and pressed Start. I was on a roll, and there was no stopping me now.

Going back upstairs to check on Mike, I collected more laundry for washing. I peeked into the bedroom and saw Mike resting comfortably, so I went back downstairs to the utility room. As I approached that room, I saw water spraying out the top of the washing machine onto the floor. With the entire utility floor flooded with water. *What happened here?* Never had this happened in the history of that machine or this utility room. *Was the comforter too oversized for my top loader?* I saw water flowing out as the filling cycle continued. I leaned over the side of the machine on one foot to stop the washing cycle. At that moment, my foot slipped out from under me on the wet floor and landed me flat on the floor, my jeans and shirt soaking up some of the water. I got up halfway and slipped again, this time falling towards the cupboards lining the opposite side of the room. My right hand and wrist jammed into the cabinets with a bang. I hoped Mike did not hear. As I was about to get up again, I realized my wrist hurt like nothing I had ever experienced.

I can't believe this just happened! Deja vu. I had the same thought that came to mind when I awoke from fainting in a public place in my college days. Scary for onlookers, it embarrassed me. No onlookers today.

What if my wrist is broken? How will I manage? I had to tell Mike. My little discussion with myself did not last long; soon, the swelling began, and so did more pain.

Mike was almost asleep when I approached the bedroom. "I had a little mishap," I started. "I slipped on some water on the utility room floor and banged my wrist into the cupboards, and now it hurts, and it's beginning to swell."

"How did you do that?"

"I am washing the comforter, which is apparently too big for the washer, and water sprayed out the top onto the floor."

"Better go get an x-ray." Mike's words reassured me. He always knew what to do. I had come to depend on him to make quick decisions.

"But then I have to leave you. Will you be OK while I'm

gone?" I hoped this would be a quick trip, with only a sprained wrist.

To the ER, I drove with one hand on the steering wheel. The young ER doctor ordered an x-ray. After the usual wait, which seemed like hours, the doctor called me back into the exam room and explained the results.

"Please tell me my wrist is not broken," I pleaded. "I have a sick husband at home; he's just a couple of days out of the hospital." The doctor shook his head.

No such luck.

"You can go upstairs in this same building to the Orthopedics office, where they will help you." That orthopedic waiting room looked more packed than the ER. *But I have a crisis here!* When I finally got to see a hand specialist, I asked, "Can I get this fixed today?"

"No, not today. The scheduling desk can tell you. Likely, it will be next week."

Orthopedists have busy schedules. The earliest my surgery could be scheduled was in four days because the weekend was upon us. In so much pain and desperate for God's help, I was now in God's waiting room.

This "timeout" focused my thoughts on God, the One just waiting for me to recognize Him in my day, in charge of everything, even my broken wrist. *"My grace is sufficient for you, for my power is made perfect in weakness...for when I am weak, then I am strong."* (2 Corinthians 12:9-10). Brought to the end of being in total control, I relinquished myself to Him.

After driving back home with my right wrist in a brace, I checked on Mike. Still under pain medication and unaware of the time, Mike was surprised I was home so soon. "Is it broken?"

"Yes, but they can't fix it till Monday." I knew Mike would not return to Mayo until later next week, so my surgery day would not interfere with his schedule.

The following Monday, my girlfriend graciously offered to drive me to the SurgiCenter and wait there during the procedure. As I sat on the hospital bed in the windowless prep room, I gowned, ready to be wheeled into the surgery suite. Suddenly, the whole place went dark.

"We've lost electricity! Sit tight," someone said. In pitch blackness, I heard people scrambling nearby.

After a few moments, someone entered the room and informed us, "A construction dig next door severed the lines to our building." Then the nurse said, "You need to get dressed. There will be no surgery today. You will be rescheduled."

Back at home, as I explained the morning's incident to Mike, a scheduler called, changing my surgical procedure to ten-thirty the following day. A few hours later, another scheduler called and changed the surgery time to five-thirty in the morning. "Emergency cases will likely preempt the ten-thirty slot," she said. "And your case could get canceled altogether." At this, I felt pity overtaking me. "Lord, I am now partially incapacitated, and Mike is totally so. Can I bear any more?" I recalled the verse, *"He will not let your foot slip—he who watches over you will not slumber"* (Psalm 121:3, NIV).

Yes, Lord, my foot slipped. Please hold me up through this, too.

At four forty-five the following morning, I took a taxi to my own surgery.

HOLY PACKETS

With my wrist pinned and in a cast, this new encumbrance complicated my life. Losing the use of my right hand hindered some things, like getting dishes out of the cupboard and helping Mike put on his tight surgery socks. My coworkers surprised me by hiring a chef to prepare a week's meals for our freezer. My colleagues felt sorry for us both in our compromised states. *God is good. Yes, the Lord is Jehovah Jireh. He provides, and at just the right moment* (Genesis 22:13-14).

One night, a week after my surgery, I walked out of the bathroom to see Mike kneeling at the foot of our bed. I had never seen him do this before. He was weeping and talking to God, but not audibly. I did not ask him what he was praying but let this holy moment stay between God and him.

"Lord, take care of him," I prayed as I disappeared back into the bathroom. I prayed for his healing, complete physical and spiritual healing. And I prayed the prayer I prayed so often, one of the fighting verses I taught my Mikey, *"No weapon formed against you shall prosper"* (Isaiah 54:17, NKJV). I wanted total protection for Mike using the power-packed Word. There was no question in my mind God is good, and He would work out good for us—even through this trial.

I found trusting God and His strength was the only strategy for us. Depending on anything else would be like leaning against a spider web. By ourselves, we were helpless, and we would fall. Wishful thinking would not do either. We had no power to fight this war on our own. But backed up with the strength of the Lord, we stood behind the most awesome Power there is, One who moves mountains. I knew He backed up the waters of the Red Sea and the Jordan River in a heap so the Israelites could cross on dry land. He raised Jesus from the dead!

I started earnestly posting verses about healing and life everywhere in the house: on the porch coffee table, on the counter by the coffee pot, and in the bathroom mirror. I wanted God's promises front and center. As I found new ones, I read them to Mike. I wanted these gems to be holy packets of comfort, strength, and hope that upheld us. And at this most fragile time, I wanted God to hold me. Mike did not yet know the gravity of his situation. He did not hear the doctor's "sorry" words. All I could do was pray and uphold us both with God's Word.

The pastor of the Stephen Ministry of our church called me and asked if he could visit. He oversaw our church's Stephen Ministry, training people for confidential Christian spiritual support and care for persons going through a crisis. Being a Stephen Minister for several years, I knew how valuable such care could be. He asked if we would like some elders to pray over Mike and anoint him with oil for healing.

"Yes, yes! Please come!"

When they arrived, I motioned for them to take chairs in our family room around Mike, draped with a blanket to cover his catheter and paraphernalia still in place from the surgery. At one end of the room, the fireplace radiated a warmth that filled the entire space. One elder read the Scripture, *"Is anyone among you sick? Let them call the church elders to pray over them and anoint them with oil in the name of the Lord"* (James 5:14, NIV). This passage talked first about asking forgiveness before we prayed for healing.

"Is there anything in your life you need to ask for forgiveness?" one elder asked Mike.

Well, everything. Both of us had repented our sinful ways earlier in our lives and accepted God's total forgiveness. But even now, we are not perfect. Constantly popping up is pride, self-rule, and at times living distant from God. Mike, however, said no to their question. Perhaps he had done all his repenting that night on his knees at the bottom of the bed. At that moment, I privately asked for forgiveness for all our offenses. The elders then anointed Mike with oil and prayed over him. Covered with the Word and prayer, this felt so right.

2

FOCUS

YEARS YET | *NOVEMBER 2007*

Mike and I had constructed our lives around our Minneapolis home, a Montana home, and a third home in Iowa, the latter purchased several years back to frequently visit my aging parents. Managing these properties became Mike's job. A few years earlier, we decided he needed to seek a reduced workload after having health issues resulting from his focus on an all-consuming medical sales career with the resultant stress. Despite this change and my demanding work schedule, our calendar was always full of activities that kept us hopping. However, we felt the brakes coming on our plans with this cancer diagnosis.

"Can we go to Montana after these follow-up appointments?" Mike asked as we sat in the consultation room, waiting for the doctor for Mike's post-surgery visit.

"I guess we can ask the doctor," I replied.

Mike and I loved Montana. I thought about when we first

considered buying that property. Mike dreamt big, things I would never consider. One of those dreams included purchasing a place in Montana. He was always one to imagine possibilities, possibilities for the present, the next week, and the future, maybe because of his earlier days without much money.

Mike grew up in Iowa and attended the local Iowa Mountaineer Club to view travel slide shows of their expeditions worldwide. In those days, he had to settle for climbing excursions to Devil's Lake, Wisconsin. But early in our marriage, he joined them for more exciting expeditions to climb mountains in the Bugaboos in Canada and Uruashraju Mountain in Peru.

I always imagined Mike had this dream compartment in his brain. When it was triggered, nothing could stand in his way. He would fight like a bulldog to achieve it. Mike was blessed with business savvy to bring such dreams to fruition. To think I was the one with a graduate business degree, but he had a business mindset. If managing our finances had been left to me, I am sure we would die with all our money intact. Not Mike! "Life is to be lived now! Enjoy it!" To him, every day was a door to a new beginning, and life was always a cup half-full. We never argued about the money for long because Mike, with his computer brain and his cover-all-arguments and negotiating skills, convinced me of the workability of his plan. He had the end game in sight.

In contrast, my more mundane approach to life included analysis, gathering data for decision-making, and pushing the pause button several times. "How can we afford that?" I said each time I saw money flying out the door. In our marriage of thirty-two years, Mike was never hesitant about spending money for new cars, clothes galore, and every imaginable piece of machinery for our Montana "ranch," as he liked to call it.

I reflected our Montana home was so unlike our home in Minnesota. Montana became our halcyon place to recoup some peacefulness. We both enjoyed that first piney scent we breathed when we opened our car door upon each arrival. There we could relax and kick back from all the happenings at home. If we arrived in July, daises would dot the meadow. In my journal, I cataloged all the other blooming plants at our property—the wild strawberry, violets, kinnikinnick, pussy-toes, and heart-leafed Arnica. I recalled Mike's favorite pastime in Montana was sitting on the deck, viewing the mountains in the Bob Marshall Wilderness.

Looking at him now, waiting for the doctor, I saw a man pondering how to live to the fullest in the present moment. Then I remembered all those mountains Mike had climbed earlier in his life in the Rockies and other places. Those were nothing compared to the cancer mountain he now faced. Planning a trip to Montana was out of our minds for a bit.

The main reason for this day's visit was to remove Mike's catheter. Unfortunately, the catheter would not come out today due to some abnormality the urologist saw on the screen. After this disappointment, Mike dressed, and we were escorted into a consultation room to wait for the doctor to tell us when the catheter could be removed. I felt so bad for Mike going through the lengthy surgery, fainting from so much blood loss, and now still tied to a catheter.

The urologist came into our little room and sat in the chair in front of his computer. He said the catheter would remain in place until the following week. He also informed us, "Of twenty-two lymph nodes removed, eight were malignant. And cancer was also found in the border of the bladder." Then he told us Mike had a particularly aggressive form of cancer when evaluated histologically. Mike's cancer cells were deemed a 9 in aggressiveness on a scale of 10, with ten being the worst.

Whoa! This news is worse than I imagined. Mike was silent, but I could tell by his deep sigh this blew him away. I pulled Mike's hand into mine and held it tight as we heard more. The doctor explained that some therapies could keep this cancer under control. At the end of his comments, he said, "You can live years yet."

Such a terrible report, yet I heard 'years yet.' A lifeline!

We hurriedly left the clinic, desperately trying to digest the doctor's contradictory statements. One painted Mike as sentenced, and the other offered hope. I attempted to cheer Mike in the car, "Did you hear that, Mikey? Years! He said you can live years yet!" I said it to shield us from the dreadful revelation we just heard.

"What does all that mean?" Mike agonized. "That the cancer has spread?" Tears flowed freely for both of us. "Why wasn't this caught earlier? Things would be so different."

I should have driven, but tears precluded my view. "Mikey, he said even though it has spread, they have therapies. It has been his experience; you have years yet!"

"Years. Does that mean ten years? Or two?"

"I don't know, but he is the expert, and he said there are treatments that can combat the progression of the cancer."

I usually emailed my sisters on the ride home after each Mayo visit, updating them on the latest news. But I could not bear to write my sisters about this outcome. The lymph nodes and bladder news stung. The two-sided pronouncement of cancer already spread outside the prostate, yet a hope Mike could 'live years' did not quell the spreading dread overtaking me. Overwhelmed by this new information from Mike's doctor, I needed time to process. Instead, this frightening news penetrated my soul, leaving me stunned.

I needed time to pray and talk with God. Where was He taking us? The "years yet" offered a ray of hope. As we arrived home from Mayo Clinic, I thought about the job I had to do: research articles defining Mike's cancer stage. I started my career in medical research, so I was familiar with locating medical literature. My goal became understanding the prognosis for Mike's type and stage of cancer. How long might Mike live?

My upstairs study room was far away from Mike's view, so in the evenings after work, I spent a little time searching for medical journal articles to give me clues about the longevity of people with this type and stage of cancer. But before understanding these articles, I had to learn the terminology, acronyms, and cancer rating systems delineated in these clinical articles.

Locating published outcome studies, some even authored by Mike's surgeon, I quickly printed them for any clues they might offer. Some articles reported statistics on large groups of metastatic prostate cancer patients addressing longevity. I knew I could not translate the calculated averages to my husband's case. His was an individual case, and his prognosis could differ widely from those averages on either end. My thoughts settled on the worst-case scenario. I also knew the gravity of the surgery results. The doctor knew the statistics. He might as well have said, "The bus has already left the station."

VALLEY OF THE SHADOW

I hunted for reassurance as Mike and I were walking through this cancer valley. I reviewed the clinical literature and learned statistics for outcomes of patients with metastatic prostate cancer. Only God could bridge us across this. On our own, we could not wrestle with this beast. I knew fighting this cancer was not our job; that was God's job. God already defeated the works of the Devil. We had only to lean on Him, His Word, even when the outlook appeared dire. I told Mike the same verse I repeated to myself, God Himself will fight for us (Deuteronomy 3:22, NKJV).

Years earlier, my stepfather, Bill, had been hospitalized with a life-threatening infection. I remember that while I was taking a shower one night, a verse came to me; "he would live and not die." I knew that was a Bible verse but did not know the reference. Researching, I found it in the Psalms. *"I will not die, but live, and will proclaim what the Lord has done"* (Psalm 118:17, NIV). I realized I declared this verse over my stepfather. He did recover, so I knew the healing power of God in my family. I pondered if Mike would be healed and we would have a long life together.

I could not keep fear out of my thinking. It kept popping up even as I repeated the Scriptures. These thoughts danced around me as if they owned me. Fear captured my emotions, too, at times. As I read the outcome studies, this cancer reality became more evident. This cancer could be an ongoing battle, a relentless struggle. The only way I knew to meet it offensively was by repeating the Scriptures as Jesus did during His wilderness experience with the Devil.

As I entered our family room, where Mike was sitting in his

recliner chair, he asked, "Where is that verse about the Word of God being alive and active?"

I couldn't remember but exclaimed, "Oh, I love that verse! It means His Word is alive and actively working right now." I told Mike the story I heard a rabbi relay from the Jewish oral history that pictures God's words as *living* words. Moses was coming down the mountain carrying the tablets of stone with words written on them by the finger of God. The words *danced* on those stone tablets.

"Yes, Mikey!" I said. "God is alive and active, and He *Himself* fights for us! Who else in this world says, 'I will fight for you?' None of the other gods people worship promise to fight for them or be with them through their struggles," I exclaimed. "What an awesome God. He not only fights for us, but He also calms our spirits. And remember, our God is the only God who forgives sins and promises the Holy Spirit within us for our daily living."

Mike and I needed God's Word to be alive and working for us. It was hard for both of us not to think about Mike's cancer diagnosis and surgery outcome. Sometimes we were like Peter, who began to walk on water. But when he took his eyes off Jesus and looked at the waves and the danger beneath him, he could no longer stay above water (Matthew 14:28-31). Like Peter, the more we focused on the problem, the more anxious we found ourselves. But when we read the living Word and focused on God, we felt calm.

I knew the Bible contains many verses that tell us, "Do not fear." Repeating those words emphasized the Lord's constant presence even in severe trials. We needed continual refocusing on God's Word and not letting our feelings reign. Our great God helped the Israelites at Migdol when they faced the approaching Egyptian army on one side and the waters on the other. They were in a tight spot, but God saved them (Exodus 14:1-3).

Please help us through this tight spot, too.

I wanted to encourage Mike, too, and told him, "For me right now, I want God's peace in our struggle. I want the peace of knowing a living and active God walks with us through this trial." I knew Mike loved to think about peace and the other fruits of the Spirit from Galatians. He had memorized them in a particular way to recall them—Love, Joy, (2 P's) Peace, Patience, (2 G's) Gentleness, Goodness, KFC: Kindness, Faithfulness, Self-Control. How he remembered the last three was *K F SChicken*.

I wanted that peace in our lives, but those daily darts of fear pierced me even as I said this. What could I do to keep them from wiping out my inner peace? I then prayed for God to take those darts, turn them around, and send them back to where they originated.

CLARITY

I continued to post "Promise Verses" on our kitchen refrigerator in our Minneapolis home. I could view them from where I sat at the center counter. This one I particularly loved: *"Surely the righteous will never be shaken; they will be remembered forever. They will have no fear of bad news; their hearts are steadfast, trusting in the Lord"* (Psalm 112:6–7, NIV).

A tiny, framed blackboard rested on the counter next to the refrigerator. On it, I copied the words I'd heard at a city-wide prayer breakfast—*Trust Me, I Got That*. A speaker at this meeting explained how these words came to him with each of several painful trials he went through after his recent conversion. During these rough times of getting back on his feet, God was saying these words to him. "Trust Me; I got that," and "Trust Me, I got you." I knew God was saying that to us, too.

Moving from the counter to my chair in the family room, I recalled how startled we had been when we heard Mike had cancer. We often heard of others around us diagnosed with cancer, but our cancer news hit us like a bomb. And this bomb never seemed to stop exploding. It left caverns right in front of us, and sometimes, we fell right into them. We noticed the world goes on, ignoring our bombed-out place. I knew we had to rely on God. He was all we had. I wanted not to be afraid or terrified of cancer.

I wish there were no such thing as cancer. Why does God allow it at all? Full of questions for God, we wondered if we were now in the furnace of affliction. Yes, *"in this world you will have trouble"* (John 16:33, NIV). We knew that verse.

Is this our test? Are we being measured by this trial?

It was so easy to question God about why this happened to us. And I knew it was okay to talk with God about our questions, even show our doubts. Yet anxiety often overtook me. This cancer thing could be growing inside of Mike. *God, is this Your best for us right now? Isn't there a better way?*

In my mind, one minute, I trusted God, and the next, I worried. *Stop this seesaw! Do I know of anything more trustworthy than the Word?* I thought of plenty of Scriptures equating the Word as truth—God-breathed. If God spoke the truth, and He does not change, and He does not lie, we can trust His promises for us, and the Word is true for us today, I reasoned.

About that time, I began reviewing for Mike one of God's attributes, His integrity. "I know God cannot go against His character. If His Word is not the truth, then He is not God with complete integrity." I went on to explain His Word is truth, total truth. The Bible states it is unmovable, and cannot be broken, undone, or annulled. It will never be void or of no effect! And so I told Mike, "Because it is the truth, we can count on all His promises for our lives. We can have total confidence in every word of His. His Word should be our solid basis going forward in persevering through this valley of ours." This basis and only this enabled me to face our new reality. We determined to rely on God's Word as truth, even if the path ahead seemed dark. We trusted the Word. We depended on it. We genuinely wanted this Word to be the focus, not the cancer problem.

HIATUS | *DECEMBER 2007*

Clinic day arrived again. We were back at Mayo Clinic for another appointment. After checking into our hotel, we walked across the street to Mayo's basement phlebotomy clinic. After giving a blood sample for testing, we searched for a new restaurant. We were tired of eating at our hotel, although the food was excellent. Even contemplating a new restaurant held no joy.

Late the next afternoon, we met with Mike's doctor. As we sat down, I recalled the last time we were here and the shocking news we'd heard. Will this just be a continuation of that news?

"I have some good news," the doctor began. "Your blood test shows you have no evidence of disease,"

"Does that mean you got all the cancer?" Mike jumped in.

Our spirits soared at once. I wanted to jump up and down

and yell, "Thank You, Lord," but contained myself. Yelling and screaming for joy would be so out of character for me. Silently, I prayed, "Thank You, Lord," and then immediately chided myself, *O, ye of little faith* to let the awful cancer news flatten me earlier.

The doctor continued, "No evidence of disease means it cannot be detected with our method of testing PSA. This test indicates you have no detectable level."

"Does this mean I am cancer-free?"

"We don't use those terms. We can only say it is below the detectable level of our method. With your cancer removed, we want that PSA number to be undetectable. Going forward, it will be a measure of any cancer cells that might be left in your body. For post-operative men for whom the cancer was all contained within the prostate gland, their number should remain undetectable because no prostate cells remain. We hope, of course, that the cancer was all removed for you as well. Do you have any questions?"

Mike looked at me. Overwhelmed by the good news, he now wanted me to take the ball and interact with the doctor, but the doctor was still looking at him.

"Well, you can think about any questions you may have, and we can talk next visit. I am recommending a therapy designed to cut the nutrition from any cancer that may be left. If you agree with my plan, you will receive this therapy today and every three months by injection. Before meeting again in three months, your blood will be checked for PSA. Does that plan sound reasonable?"

"Let's do it," Mike exclaimed, entirely on board.

"The nurse will give you your first injection right after we finish."

He explained how with every drug, there are side effects. The only one that registered was fatigue. *That doesn't sound too bad.* I had read those clinical articles about this drug but had not paid attention to the side effects. My focus was on outcomes and prognosis.

SEVEN TIMES | *WINTER 2007*

As Mike regained strength, I looked for prayer and support everywhere. I found the Healing Rooms of St. Paul online. I had read about John G. Lake, a minister whom God used for great healing miracles in the Spokane area in the early 1900s. There he established Healing Rooms and demonstrated the power of God in healing thousands of people. I read he would go into the Spokane hospital and pray for the sick and clear the place of patients.

Since our Montana home was not so far from Spokane, I envisioned making a trip to the Healing Rooms. But unfortunately, I knew we would not be going to Montana soon because of follow-up doctor appointments. So, I approached the idea of going to the Healing Rooms near us in St. Paul, to which Mike emphatically replied, "Yes, definitely! Let's go."

I found the address of the Healing Rooms near us. In a modest building, we waited in a small lobby room, checking out the reading materials they displayed on tables. We were open to God working a miracle for Mike if that was His plan. Two people came to meet us and led us into another room, relatively empty except for a chair in the center of the room. They listened to Mike's story about his diagnosis, surgery, and recovery thus far. We asked for prayer for his healing. After

I'M GOING TO RUN UNTIL I'M DONE

praying for Mike, they wanted us to take some literature from the lobby. We left feeling peace over us.

Back home, we settled into our family room. With our sun porch closed for the winter months, Mike sat silently in his recliner facing the brick fireplace and TV. Before his diagnosis, he was in the best shape of his life, even at age sixty-one. His running log included days of running long mileages, sometimes up to nine miles a day. This cancer fit into none of our plans. We sometimes felt blindsided and shortchanged, even hobbled by our new reality.

Like enduring the agony of "hitting the wall" at mile 20—the well-known wall of pain marathoners experience when muscle glycogen becomes depleted—Mike took on this new challenge. He was not about to let this unwelcome chapter affect him without a fight. His brother-in-law, Dan, did not call him Iron Mike without reason. Mike thought nothing of chopping wood at our Montana home or working in the forest for hours at a stretch. Physical challenges were part of his DNA. Beginning in his youth, Mike was a serious runner before running was even in vogue. He ran seven and eight miles a day when I first met him. He owned the first-generation Nike Air Jordan running shoes.

Mike maintained this steely determination in all his outdoor activities. Some of that grit came from playing college golf, competing in tournaments against some tough players of his day who later became regulars on the pro-golf circuit—Ben Crenshaw, John Mahaffey, and Johnny Miller. Mike's climbing journal recorded the "fourteeners" and classic peaks he climbed in Colorado—Mount Bierstadt, Mount Sniktau, Grizzly Peak, Grays Peak, Kelso, Mount Bross, Lincoln, Democrat, Sherman,

Brow, Huron, Lady McDonald, Torreys, Granite Peak, Audubon, Evans, Quandary Peak, Pikes Peak, Lady Washington, Chiefs Head Peak, Pawnee Peak, Mount Orton, Warbonnet Peak, and Long's Peak. Most of the Colorado mountains he climbed alone. On trips with the Iowa Mountaineers, he climbed the Sawtooths in Idaho, the Bugaboos, Mount Athabasca, Eiffel Peak in British Columbia, and Aconcagua in Argentina. Mike knew what physical endurance meant. In addition, his ability to "zone in" became integral to how he conquered goals. Competition egged him on, and tenacity seemed to be his second name. These traits were visible in all areas of his life, including being the number one salesman in several medical products companies.

Personal challenges were no stranger to him, either. For Mike, they seemed to occur with regularity. The first major hit came in his high school days when his parents divorced. He felt abandoned, even orphaned, he said. There had been bad experiences in the home, too, with alcoholism and abuse. When both of his parents died young, Mike felt even more abandoned.

Then his previous marriage fell apart after a few short years. Much later, health issues arose—ankylosing spondylitis and now prostate cancer. Rough periods were strewn across his life, knocking Mike blow after blow. We recognized how the hand of God had been over Mike's life and how his grandmother Nana's covering prayers were still in effect. Nana, always smiling with wispy white hair piled up in a bun, had bulldog faith, holding Mike up through each trial.

As we sat in our family room, a peacefulness settled over us that we wanted to savor for the moment.

Mike finally broke the silence. "Could God heal me of cancer?"

"Your life and what has happened to you reminds me of a verse in Proverbs," I answered, "*'for though a righteous man falls seven times, he rises again.'*" God saw you through all of your previous blows. He will see you through this one, too. Let's pray that He will. You know the truth of the Bible trumps facts."

BUOYED | *MARCH 2008*

Three months went by quickly, and spring arrived. Mike, healed from his surgery, began his running routine again. Attitude-wise, his spirits were upbeat. Watching him return to his old self, I pondered the goodness of God as I sat on our sunny, heated porch, taking in the warmth and beauty of the early spring day. I saw Mike's humor return. On the spot, he would invent new words out of old ones, like describing the changeable weather in Minnesota as *spritzophrenic* or *artic-apolis*.

As I considered that we would be traveling back to Mayo Clinic for another checkup, a bit of anxiety slipped in when contemplating the unknown results of Mike's next blood test. These doctor appointments arrived like clockwork, reminding us we were not in charge. I had to relinquish that into God's hands and not hold the reins so tightly. It became a moment-by-moment process. When my soul told me to be worried, my spirit told me to *"be anxious for nothing"* (Philippians 4:6).

Arriving early at the clinic, we proceeded to the basement blood-drawing area. Mike's blood-test results, needed by the doctor to determine Mike's status, would be available by the late afternoon appointment. While waiting, we visited the shops around Mayo Clinic and then had lunch at the Greek deli across the street. In the afternoon, we walked back to the

Landow Atrium and joined a room full of other patients who quietly waited for their appointments. Music played softly in the background, intended to ease any stress. I hated the drama of this all-day waiting, coming early for blood tests, then waiting till four o'clock to hear the results. Waiting all day for just a few words to answer the question: Is the cancer controlled?

Taking the elevator up to the eighth floor, we soon arrived at our clinic. Finally, four o'clock came, and they called Mike's name. The nurse took us into a small consultation room, a familiar routine. There we waited on pins and needles to hear the blood test results.

As the doctor entered, I could not discern from his countenance whether he had good news or bad. *He'd make a good poker player.*

"No tumor marker is evident," he said. "It is under the detectable level; there is no evidence of disease."

Yes! I call that praise! This fantastic news pushed me to think about what God was orchestrating in our lives. I found it hard to concentrate on anything else the doctor said. He asked about how Mike was doing. Mike talked about the loss of stamina and decreased ability to run as far or as fast. Mike wanted to know about hot flashes that were becoming more evident. These negatives seemed reasonable to me, as long as the quarterly injections could control the cancer.

All the way home, we praised God profusely for staving off this aggressive cancer. *We have the God who heals all our diseases! All is copacetic. Mike is not dying; he is going to live. With God, nothing is impossible!* We immediately relayed the good news to family and friends via emails, with all praise given to God. With this answer to prayer, Mike would have a reprieve from this dreadful invader. *God is in charge. God is working in Mike's life, all by His grace.*

I called Mike my Miracle Man, not just because of the clinic's good news we'd just received. He was a Miracle Man before this, too. A decade earlier, God graciously removed Mike's ankylosing spondylitis pain overnight with a new designer drug. The following day, after his first dose, we sat on our porch, laughing and praising the God who heals. All of Mike's pain and symptoms were completely gone forever. The rheumatologist said Mike could be the poster boy for this drug. We knew, of course, that the Lord had healed him. After this miracle, Mike even ran two more marathons! So, we knew the God who heals and that He could handle this cancer problem, too.

After this celebration, I exclaimed, "Can this get any better?"

RERUN | *2008-2009*

Over the next couple of years, we heard, again and again, the excellent result of Mike's blood tests—"no evidence of disease." Mike used opportunities to tell people his cancer story, how he had no evidence of disease, even with late-stage cancer. God was with him through this struggle. Initiating conversations with strangers came easy for him. He talked with anyone he met, including clerks at the grocery store, coffee shops, neighbors, repairmen, and even people he met at gas stations. He asked them if they knew anyone who had cancer. Of course, everyone did. He then told them his cancer story and counted on God for his life. Then he gave them the laminated brochure, *God's Promises for Hope and Courage*. He indicated they should give that brochure to the cancer patient they had mentioned, knowing they would look at it themselves. I had to reorder those brochures several times to have enough on hand. He wanted his acquaintances to know the God who heals and helps him.

Mike kept up his running schedule, albeit reduced in distance and increased in time. Clocking himself, he recorded the length and time of his Luce Line route in his daily running log. On this jogging path, as people passed him, Mike would say, "Can't run faster than a cancer man." He made people stop to talk to him, and when they did, he told them his cancer story. People were amazed he could run with metastatic cancer. They seemed open to listening to him because he represented someone in the struggle of his life, yet he had the perseverance to go on.

Mike told me of one runner, an attorney named Tim, whom Mike often met on the Luce Line Trail. It must have been one of those first times that Mike told Tim his cancer story and how God had blessed him with good cancer reports. After that, Mike said Tim never failed to stop and pray over Mike right there on the trail.

As Mike met people, they would tell him of a family member who had cancer. Mike collected these names and added them to a growing list of over thirty people for whom he prayed daily. He memorized their names in a particular order and repeated them in his prayer each morning. Mike prayed they all would come to know the Lord. He wanted each of them to meet the One who gave him so much peace. He wanted them all "to just get this right," as he'd said to his nephew, Andy, who was dying of cancer. Mike did not want anyone to miss the opportunity to believe in the Lord, have their sins forgiven, and have eternal life. I, too, wanted Andy to know the Father's great love to provide His Son as a sacrifice to pay for our sins. No earning and deserving required, just believing and receiving. He could experience "new" life with God.

As Mike continued his daily runs, he realized this new drug sapped his strength and energy. He could not go as fast or far on the trail as before. I noticed his restlessness and his disturbed sleep. "I feel half-sick sometimes, and what are all these hot flashes?" Mike wanted to know. As fear showed its face again, I looked for "Do not fear" verses and peppered the kitchen counters and our mirrors with them, so they were never far from view. While others placed their trust solely in doctors and wishful thinking, I tried to elevate our thinking with the Word. I continued to tell Mike we were adopted children of God. He promises He is with us continually. He never abandons us.

I needed to reiterate this truth to myself. "Even when we do not always feel God's closeness," I said, "the Word says He is right there beside us, always working. Remember what the name *Immanuel* means? God with us. He patiently waits for us to recognize His Presence."

I realized I needed to rely on God's Word, not my feelings, to be my source of strength and hope. It became my anchor, solidifying my focus for the road ahead.

ANOTHER | *MAY 2010*

Deep in concentration at work in early May, my desk phone rang and jarred me back to the real world. I leaned back in my chair, welcoming a break from that morning's work. I became a pro at drowning out the ubiquitous cubicle buzz around me.

Sometimes, interruptions gave me a fresh perspective when I returned to work. The call was from Mike. He had just arrived home from his yearly dermatology check-up at Mayo Clinic.

He blurted out, "They said I have malignant melanoma on my earlobe."

"What?" I exclaimed loudly.

"Yes, the doctor said a spot needs to come off."

"I can't believe this! Here you have one cancer and now another one?"

I realized everyone around me had heard the news. So I quickly moved closer to my desk and lowered my voice so our conversation would be more muffled. I had expected a routine check-up. That was not the case; now, we had to deal with two cancers.

After that news, I could not focus on work, so I drove home to be with Mike. We needed to digest this new information. "God, help," I cried on the way home. I could not believe my Mikey had another cancer diagnosis. "How are we to think about this, Lord? Isn't one cancer enough?" I recalled how a person from my childhood church had visited my brother in Arizona when he battled renal cancer. He relayed she had battled four different cancers in her adult life.

This new cancer is serious stuff. I was grasping for anything to help explain this new invasion into our lives. My mind leaped into questioning whether the two cancers were linked. In the next few weeks, I went into my research mode, scouring clinical literature for clues. I located a study by researchers from the University of Michigan and Sloan Kettering studying the various types of prostate cancer. I emailed the University of Michigan researcher to inquire about any connection between prostate and malignant melanoma cancers.

Unlike me, Mike took this new cancer interruption in stride. Maybe he could not deal with it, or perhaps he had less fear than I did at that moment, but he just went with the flow, but I was shocked at this news. In a couple of weeks, Mike said, he would have surgery. The doctor described how they would cut off that earlobe and replace it with a new earlobe constructed from skin taken from Mike's neck.

Surgery day came. Mike was under some but not total anesthesia, and as the doctor worked, I was allowed to be in the room but distanced from the surgery area. Mike talked the entire time. When he came out of the anesthesia, Mike asked the surgeon, "How did it go?"

"Just fine. I reconstructed your earlobe. It will be hard to tell this is not your original earlobe."

"Did I do OK?"

"You did fine. You talked a lot."

"I hope I didn't say anything revealing or out of line."

"No, you talked the entire time about golf. Are you a golfer?" Mike explained that he was once a professional golfer and would soon go to a golf reunion of old college buddies.

After Mike's release from recovery, someone wheeled him to the Mayo Clinic canopy entrance, where I met him with the car to drive home. On the way home, Mike told me that he heard the scissors snip his earlobe during the surgery. *That audible snip certainly did not phase his continual one-sided golf conversation.*

Mike's love of golf started early with new golf clubs from his mother. His father did not want to spend the money, but his mother did it anyway. Since Mike's family lived close to Finkbine Golf Course in Iowa City, he played daily, if not several times a day. He worked at the club, so the management allowed him to play the course when no one else was playing.

He began winning local tournaments and prizes in high school and ranked high in the Midwest among players, which led to a full-ride golf scholarship to Eastern New Mexico University. From his first year, Mike was a varsity player. When a former team member contacted him about a golf reunion, Mike told him of his cancer situation and said he could only attend if his wife also came. I knew that Mike, in his fatigued state, needed my support to attend after this second cancer diagnosis.

That August, the former team members gathered at an Italian restaurant in Des Moines. As I ate my pasta, I listened to the guys reminiscing about tournaments, shots, stories, and jokes; they said they kept it clean for me. They roared at Mike's imitation of their beloved coach, B. B., and they could not understand why Mike did not continue in golf. "You had the sweetest swing. Effortless power," one of them said. Captured in a group photo, I never saw Mike smile as widely as I did at this dinner. For a few moments, he forgot his dilemma, his new dual diagnosis.

WHOLENESS | *JULY 2011*

Despite Mike's fatigue and hot flashes, the PSA test results continued to show "no evidence of disease." Working thirty-plus years, I took early retirement to devote my full time to supporting Mike. Because I loved my work, this posed a difficult decision. Over the years, I considered my positions a perfect fit for me. They provided great satisfaction in elevating patients' quality of life. However, over the years, I had traveled extensively, and with time away from home, it became more worrisome for Mike. In the last years before I retired, he would casually ask when I would quit work. He did not push it, just a subtle suggestion. So when we heard about Mike's late-stage cancer diagnosis, I had to consider how much time he really had left.

Still in good health otherwise, Mike recovered nicely from ear surgery with no further issues. Running in several local races, Mike did not run to beat any time but to stay in the game. Elated by my retirement decision, he could not wait to spend weeks at our Montana home, even months at a time. Situated in the Swan Valley between the Mission Mountains and Swan peaks, our hideaway was the perfect place to relax. With a valley elevation of 3,600 feet, we could view Van's Peak to the east, and behind it towered Swan Peak at 9,200 feet. Trees galore populated the place: Douglas fir, spruce, ponderosa pine, larches, and lodgepole pine. With little wind in this area, the trees towered high, some even seventy and eighty feet. So thick with trees, we had no idea of the hill on the backside of the property when we purchased the place. Off the beaten path, it offered discovery and delight. It gave us a sense of place and permanence with treasures and many memories, elevating our spirits each time we visited. Loving the outdoors and adventure, we mixed just enough conveniences in this secluded place to make it our kickback place. That was easy for Mike to do. It always took me a few days after we arrived to relax and appreciate the peacefulness of the home.

In September, we settled in for a month-long stay. During this low-key trip, I grappled with all the things we had been through since Mike's prostate cancer diagnosis. I wrestled with how we should think about healing. I knew Jesus healed many people. The disciples healed people. Was healing from a dreaded disease like cancer for our day and age? My stepfather was healed of his serious infection. Mike's ankylosing spondylitis symptoms were entirely gone, all by God's grace. I witnessed healing for myself when a woman I was mentoring was healed of an autoimmune disease that had partially disabled her for several years. I knew God designed our bodies in such a way as to recover from wounds and bruises. *Would God heal Mike of cancer?*

On our Montana deck, we enjoyed the warming sun. These were the days we would spend dreaming about all winter long. Mike seemed relaxed, so I tested the waters to discuss healing. "Sickness and disease are part of this world. After the fall of man in the Garden of Eden, our world became broken. But I know God desires us to thrive, depending on Him."

He listened.

"Isaiah says, *"He Himself bore our sicknesses, and He carried our pains . . . and we are healed by His wounds"* (Isaiah 53:4–5, HCSB). By His suffering and death, He also carried our sicknesses. So, Mikey, we have His Word to come against the enemy's plan."

"Does this mean that I can be completely healed?" Mike asked.

"I do know this is true. Jesus healed in His day, and He is the same yesterday, today, and forever, so I believe in healing today. My understanding of the word *shalom* is complete wholeness—spiritually, physically, and in our whole being. That is what God desires for us."

My personal goal had been and continued to be in persistent prayer for Mike's healing, bringing to God what He said in

His Word. Even with these questions, I remembered, He would never leave us stranded, even in this worst of all trials. We were in His care. We needed that covering right now.

So I prayed:

Dear Father,

You are our Creator, the Author of our lives, and Redeemer of our souls. You are the Healer, and You are the Healing. For this, I am thankful. I am humbled as I bow before You right now. You said in Your Word, I must first cleanse my heart of any unforgiveness before I pray for healing. Right now, I forgive those who have wronged me; I forgive them now. And for holding a ledger account of offenses, cleanse me of all wrongs. All the wrong ways I went. Forgive my self-rule, my distance from You, and for thinking I can do life by myself. I give these up right now to You, the Lord Almighty, all-wise, who knows better than me what is best for our lives.

Your Word says the prayer of a righteous person is powerful and effective. I turn to You now and repeat back to You the promises of Your Word about healing. Your Word is Your power! Your Word is alive and active! As I speak these truths, I am speaking LIFE according to Your Word.

You forgive all our sins and heal all our diseases. You took up our infirmities and carried our diseases. By Your wounds, Mike is healed. You heal the brokenhearted and bind up our wounds. You send forth Your Word, and it heals us; You declare You will restore us to health and heal our wounds. Mike will not die but live and will proclaim what You have done. We will not let Your words out of our sight; we will keep them within our hearts, for they are life and health to us.

You are the Lord, the God of all creation. Is anything too hard for You? Your will be done on earth as it is in heaven. You said, "Ask, and you will receive, and my joy will be complete." Be merciful to me, Lord, for I am faint; O Lord, heal us. I know You are a refuge for the oppressed, a stronghold in times of trouble. Those who know Your name will trust in You, for You, Lord, have never forsaken those who seek You. I ask in faith, nothing wavering, for without faith, it is impossible to please You. I come to You and believe You exist, and You reward those who earnestly seek You. I now bow to You, sovereign God. Your will be done. It is in Your great name, I pray.

Amen

PLANS | OCTOBER 2011

Mike continued to hear the good news of 'no evidence of disease.' Spending extended time in the late summer in Montana, we used that time to keep up the place and prepare for the winter. We had plenty of time to enjoy and reflect on God's goodness to us. Then I considered another idea. With Mike's continued status of no evidence of disease, I said, "Let's do something different. How about a trip to Israel? Wouldn't that be the trip of a lifetime? We can do a short one, so you won't be too tired."

"Ok, but plan it so I can rest at times."

"I'll look online to see if there is a way we can go for a week. Would you be up for that?"

"Yes, I suppose." I thought I could plan a self-directed trip, maybe get a tour guide for several days and spend the rest of the time by ourselves in Jerusalem. But unfortunately, I found only eleven-day tour group plans on my computer. That was too long for Mike. Then I remembered our church took trips to

Israel, so I called our church. The woman who answered the phone indicated they had a tour group next March, and I should contact the coordinator. I quickly learned they had already filled their quota, except two people had canceled just that day.

"Excellent!" I said. "Mark us in." Then I explained my husband had cancer and would need rest times.

"No problem. Your husband can rest in the hotel room on days when he is not feeling well." Done! We booked the trip. Excitement filled us. We were going to Israel.

The following week, we flew home from Montana. Upon arrival in Minneapolis, I received a call from my sister saying my ninety-seven-year-old mother was in the hospital and not doing well. I needed to see her. I quickly gathered some things and drove the 270 miles to the Iowa hospital. When I arrived at her hospital room, I could see she was not talking much and was quite restless.

My mind rushed to a conclusion—she could be dying. When the doctor said he was keeping her as comfortable as possible but not taking any heroic measures, all my thoughts zoomed in on losing her. She was the backbone of our family and held us together, my pillar. I counted on her continual prayers to cover Mike and me.

I telephoned Mike. "This does not look good," I said. "She may not last long. The doctor is keeping her comfortable. I am going to stay a few days, but I will be home for your appointment." Several years earlier, Mike had written my mother a love letter, telling her how much he appreciated her strength, love, and her continual prayers for us. Now it became our turn to pray for her and support her through this chapter.

I reserved the community room in the nursing home as my

bedroom for my stay. At the same time, I could visit my stepfather in the nursing home. Not always convivial, I still persevered in praying for him, that someday he might become a believer.

My sister indicated she could come in a few days. As I sat by my mother's hospital bed, I pondered all our hour-long phone conversations every Saturday morning, cherishing that continuity.

The nurse said they were trying to keep my mother comfortable. Quiet most of the time and only talking when I asked a question, I could see she was very ill. I told her I was there and that I loved her. I let her know of my sister's visit in a few days. Not sure she heard me. I talked anyway. All the while, my agonizing heart wrenched to think I might be losing her.

As I continued my one-sided conversation, I thought about how strong she had been, although tiny in stature. She held up through her first husband's death (my father), leaving her with four small children to raise. When my brother died in his early fifties, she again rose to shepherd the family through that trauma. I knew her deep abiding faith pulled her through all those trials. I thanked God for her life, her witness, her caring, and her mainstay support, but my heart ached because she seemed nearly lifeless.

The third day of my stay arrived, and I had to return to Minneapolis. I promised Mike I would be back for his doctor's appointment. As I wrestled with staying and going, I knew Mike needed me, too.

I leaned over my mother's bed and whispered, "I am leaving now. I have to get back to Minneapolis to go with Mike to the doctor."

As I quietly tiptoed out of her hospital room, I heard her

clear voice from across the room, and I froze in my steps. Her voice was not loud, but her words rang out across that room. "See you in heaven."

I broke into tears; I barely spilled out, "Yes, I'll see you in heaven." My choked-up voice revealed my heart. I rushed to her side, but she had retreated.

I tried to hide my sobbing as I walked past the lobby and down the corridor towards the parking lot, but tears clouded my vision. Sitting in my car sobbing, I cried, "She is going, isn't she?" For several minutes, I was unable to drive.

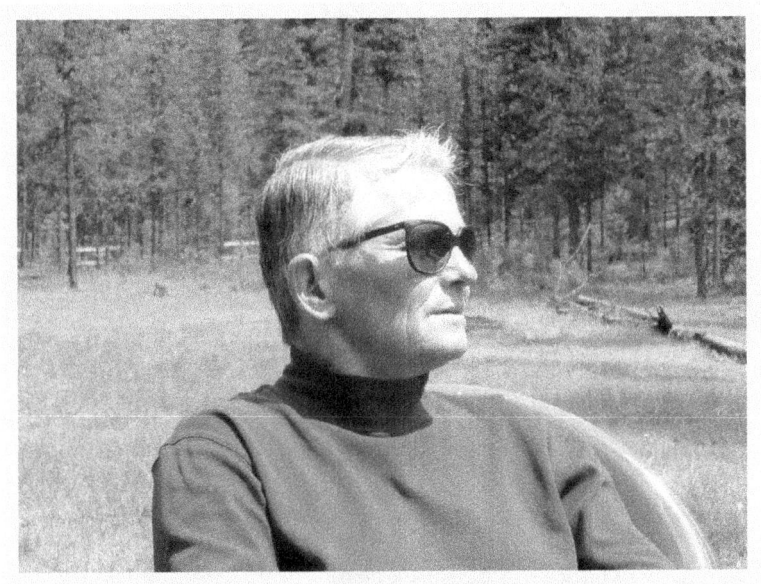

Mike at the Montana "ranch"

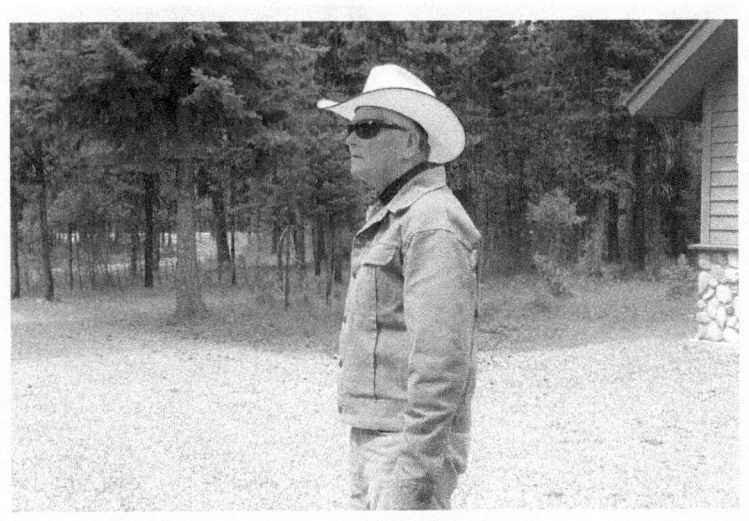

Cowboy at heart

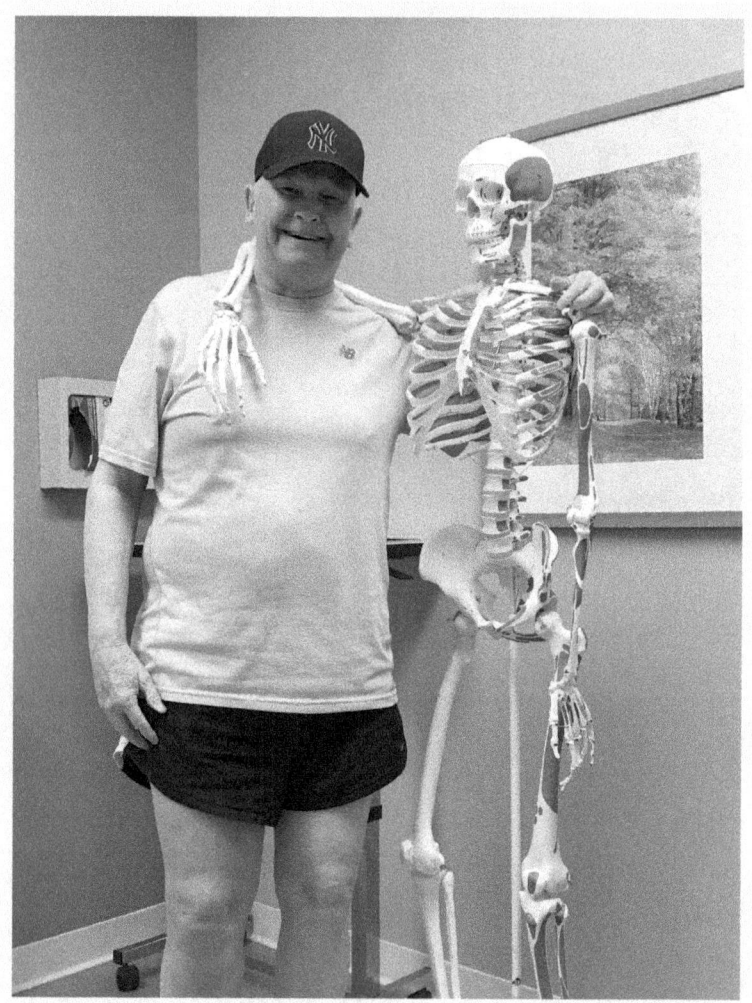

Levity in the doctor's office

I'M GOING TO RUN UNTIL I'M DONE

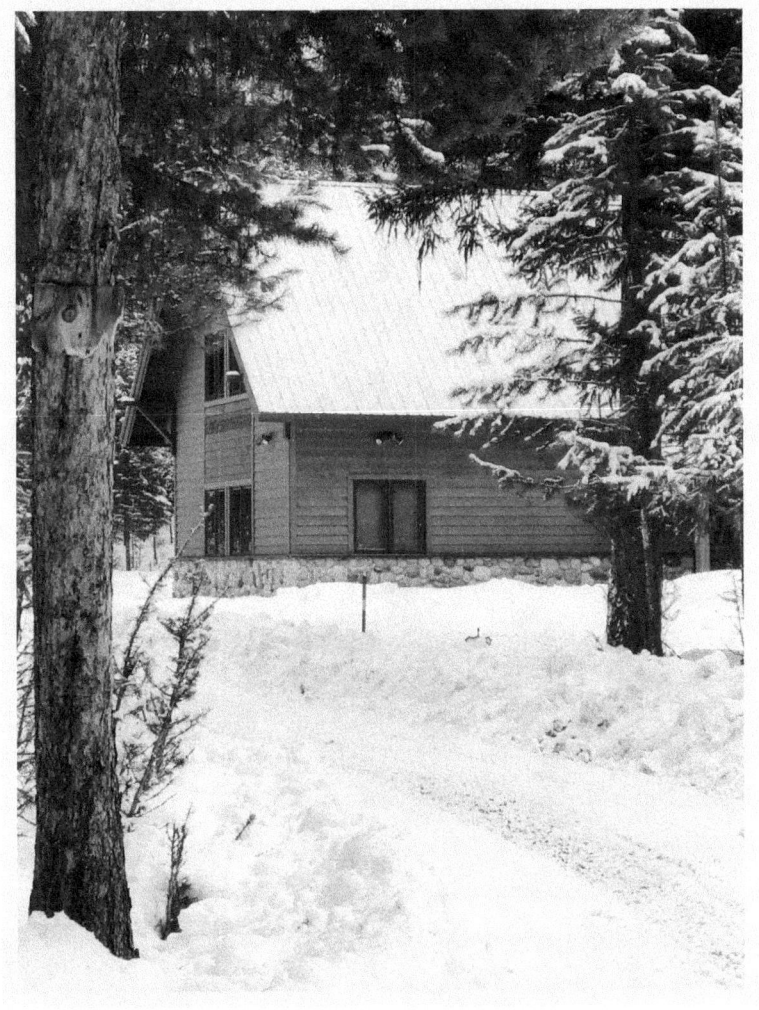

Montana cabin

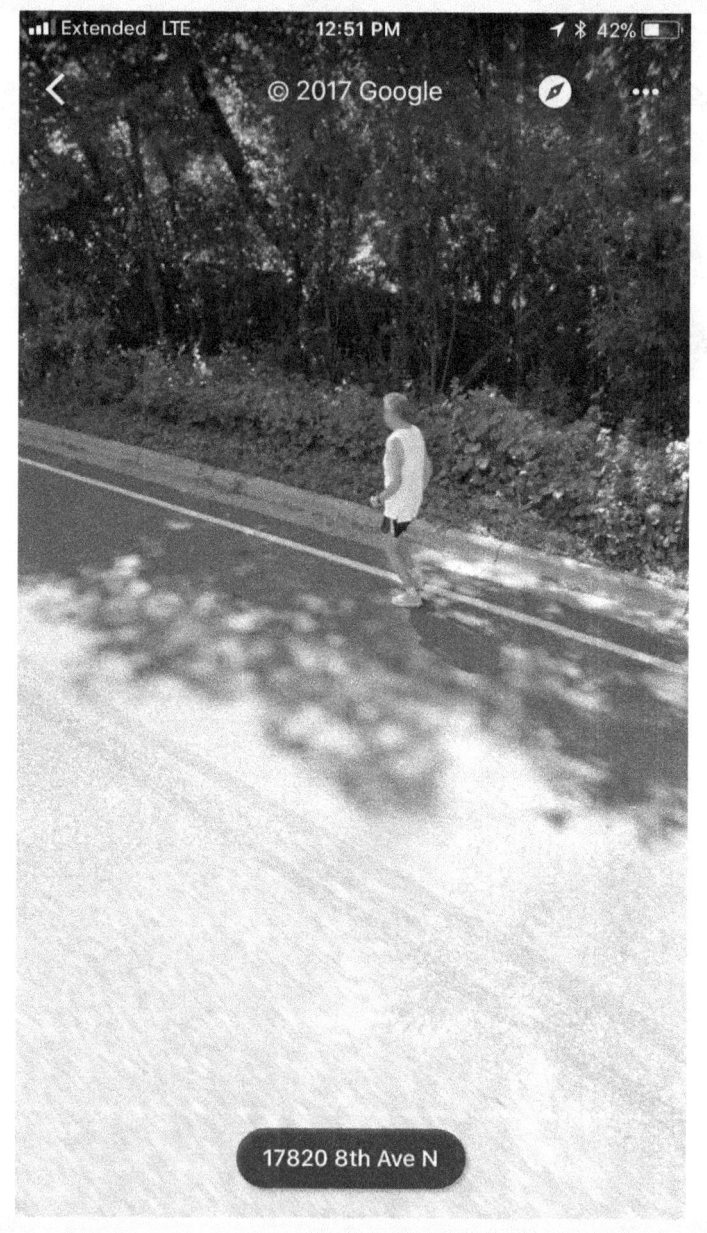

One of Mike's last runs captured on Google Earth on a street near our Minnesota home.

3
CHANGES (STILL RUNNING)

TRIP | *MARCH 2012*

Sitting at my kitchen table on a Saturday morning, I heard a pair of geese squawking as they flew low over our house, heading for the marsh just west of our home near Minneapolis. It had been months since my mother's passing. That loss punctured my thoughts. If I could talk with her, I would review the sequence of events since Mike's diagnosis. And I would relay the hope that perhaps Mike would beat the odds and live ten years after his diagnosis. That would be a miracle! *Our times are in Your hands, Lord.*

We loved the "no evidence of disease" reports we heard every three months. As I looked over the marsh, I thanked God for all He had done. We had done none of it. It was all God.

Mike came home from running that morning; he told me he had met a running acquaintance, a urologist, who told him, at some point, the cancer could mutate—finding a way around his therapy. I wanted to keep that doctor's "pronouncement" at bay and not let it play with our minds. Resolute, both Mike and I continued standing on God's Word.

Later that month, we flew to Israel for the eleven-day trip planned. Although weak, Mike trudged with the group each day to sites we never dreamed of seeing in our lifetime—places where Jesus walked and taught. Our Israeli tour guide, Ahron, a Messianic Jew, gave each site's history and biblical background. So rich were the teachings and the experience of being there we did not think about our safety in that guarded land. And for most of our waking hours, we pushed our cancer situation far back in our minds.

In Israel, we had the joy of being remarried by our pastor at the traditional Cana marriage site, the site where Jesus performed his first miracle of turning water into wine. Later both Mike and I were baptized in the Jordan River. One day, as Mike and I exited our hotel to board the tour bus, Mike strode up to our pastor and asked, "Now that you have married me and baptized me, would you also do my funeral?"

Taken aback by this request, our pastor replied, "Yes, but I hope that is a long way in the future." At that time, he was unaware Mike was sick.

NEW | *SEPTEMBER 2012*

My mother, whom I deeply missed, was gone. However, I still traveled to Iowa to visit Bill, my stepfather, in a care facility in my small hometown. He wanted a ninety-fifth birthday party, so he asked my sisters and me to plan a cake and ice cream celebration. Such a function was so unlike him. We knew him as a strongly opinionated man, but not a talkative one. We had prayed for him our whole lives that he would become a believer; years had passed, and now he was old.

My sisters and I traveled our separate ways to Iowa to plan this party. I hated leaving Mike in Minneapolis, but he decided he was not up for this event. My sisters and I carried out Bill's specific plans for the food and celebration. We invited all the nursing home residents and staff, his brother and wife, and others. We knew if we did not do it the way Bill wanted, we would hear from him. Bill indicated he wanted to speak at his celebration. Because he was a man of few words, this surprised us.

The nursing home staff wheeled Bill into their bright, sunny dining room on the afternoon of his birthday. The room quickly filled as the nursing home staff wheeled in the other residents, some overflowing into the adjoining room—the other staff filtered in, lining the bright yellow walls. With everyone situated, I welcomed them and told them Bill wanted to say a few words before we served the cake and ice cream. We had no idea what he would say. I thought he would talk about his past from his autobiography, which he hand-wrote in preparation for an obituary.

Instead, in a commanding voice from his wheelchair, Bill announced he was a believer in Jesus Christ as his Savior. He even quoted a scripture verse. My mouth dropped open. Speechless, my sisters and I sat stunned. Before us was the same man we had prayed for all those years, hoping he would become a believer. Instead of attending church back then with us, he stayed home and read the Sunday paper.

It was then that I realized the fulfillment of the rest of that verse I prayed for him so many years ago when he was in the hospital. *"I will not die, but live, and will proclaim what the Lord has done"* (Psalm 118:17, NIV). On his ninety-fifth birthday, we celebrated not only his chronological birthday but also his spiritual birthday. *Mom will really be surprised to see him in heaven.*

Before driving home to Minneapolis, I telephoned Mike. "You won't believe what happened at that party."

"Oh, no, something bad?"

"Something good! Bill announced he was a believer," I exclaimed. "You know what that shows? We should keep praying and never give up. All those years of praying for him! Who knows what God has in store for us."

SHIFT | *OCTOBER 2012*

The time for another check-up and blood draw arrived. Earlier in May, we had flown to Montana. Staying for a couple of months, we had to arrange for Mike's chemo injection to be done by a urology clinic in Missoula. At that clinic, Mike received another opinion about his injections in the last five years. This urologist explained that 'no evidence of disease' could mean he was in remission and no longer needed this drug. The only way to know was if Mike went off the medication and his PSA remained undetectable. That sounded wonderful to Mike since he had experienced so many side effects from that drug. For the first time, we envisioned that Mike could be off the medication that depleted his energy level and caused hot flashes and weight gain.

We flew home from that trip with new hope. We chose a new urologist closer to home than the Mayo Clinic. The two-day drama of driving to Mayo Clinic and waiting until the second afternoon to hear test results was too much stress for us. Choosing a urologist in an adjacent suburb, we could be there in fifteen minutes and wait a half-hour for the results. So I made the appointment.

The month came for the first visit with the new doctor. Cautiously optimistic, we traveled the short distance from our home to this clinic. They said we would hear the results of Mike's blood test in about twenty minutes. As we sat in the waiting room, the thoughts in our minds were that the results would be "no evidence of disease," as were those for the last five and half years. When we were called back into the exam room with the doctor, we were expectant that the good results would continue. I wanted the very best for Mike.

"Your test results show the PSA is slightly elevated above the detectable level."

"How much?" Mike queried.

"A tiny bit, but detectable by our test."

"Could your testing method be different than Mayo Clinic's?" I asked.

"I highly doubt that." The doctor wanted another test in three months to confirm the results.

I knew it would be hard to wait.

ADJUST | *WINTER 2013*

With the new unwanted test result, our escape was always Montana. This season Mike and I traveled by train to Whitefish, Montana, and from there to our place. We had spent most Christmases at our Montana home, delighting in the winter wonderland.

I wondered if we needed a change of vacation sites to a different place, perhaps in the summer. We had been to San

Francisco separately, earlier in our twenties, before we knew each other. Mike had escaped to a friend's place after his divorce, and I just needed a vacation from work. Neither of us had seen many sights on those trips. Being a former hiker and mountain climber, Mike wanted to see Yosemite. I just wanted new scenery, a getaway. Yes, Montana was grand, but seeing someplace different, I thought, would perk up our lives, which had become one doctor visit after another interspersed with trips to Montana.

As we reviewed places we wanted to see, we settled on a trip in the late summer. I selected a package deal for the flight and hotel and tacked on a San Francisco bus tour and a bus tour to Yosemite. With the bus tours, we would not have to walk to see sights, and Mike would not be exhausted.

Satisfied that we had some getaway plans for the following summer, we settled into watching the Superbowl when the phone rang. I knew coming out to Montana posed some challenges. My stepfather, Bill, had been declining in recent months. I told the nursing home to call me if his status changed. That night we learned of his death. Turning off the TV, we were quiet, considering what we should do. Located seventy-five miles from the train station, I immediately felt the urge to leave. As Bill's power of attorney and now his executor, I had to get organized.

I quickly changed our train tickets and asked our neighbors to take us to the train station at Whitefish. On the two-day train trip home, we watched the landscape change from mountains to plains. Mike rested most of the time. I needed quiet time to reflect on this happening—Bill's homegoing. I made calls to the funeral home and the extended family. Without interruption, I could spend hours on those plans from our private sleeping compartment. All I could think to say was, "Yay, Lord! How You turn things for Your good. Bill is with You now."

MARCH 2013

With the funeral behind us, we focused on Mike's next three-month appointment. Waiting for the next test result was agonizing. I prayed the previous test result was a fluke within the variation of the test.

When the appointment day finally came, Mike became slightly agitated. "Let's get this over!" He wanted the blood draw and twenty-minute waiting period for the test results to get over fast, not that he had any plans that day except running. He took off his jacket at the clinic and bared his arm for the blood draw. Then we sat down in the waiting room for what seemed an interminably long time.

Churning inside, I pondered the possible results ahead of us while pleading, *Please, God, bring us the good news that the last test results were not real.*

Mike jumped up. "I'm going to walk around outside." This drama rattled me, just like waiting for test results at Mayo. The results could either be good or bad. Had the last test just been a fluke, or was it real? I wondered. I did not know. I just prayed for calm because the anxiety inside me flooded to the surface.

Mike came back into the waiting room, and finally, the doctor called us back into the room.

"Your PSA is up just a little more. Not much, but a little."

"Now, what?" Mike wanted to know.

"Well, I would like to have you back on the same injection. We can give it here today."

What other choice did we have? Mike did not want to go back on that drug. But now, his PSA was climbing. The doctor convinced him to go back on the therapy.

I prayed all the way home for another option, but I knew we were probably turning a corner. *Where are You taking us, Lord?* Those words about mutation from the running friend we wanted to forget now demanded attention. That day Mike wrote in his running journal, "BAD! BAD! BAD! BAD DAY!

HOPE | *SPRING 2013*

Back home from that appointment, Mike said he was going running. I saw how Mike's therapy left him listless and played havoc with his metabolic and hormonal systems, but his intrepid spirit carried him forward. He persevered, running most days. He did not run fast; some people walked faster than he ran. Undaunted, he was determined to stay fit, either on the Luce Line or the treadmill, despite his depleted energy condition. Every single run, he recorded in his running log. Mike once wrote a note I found on our porch coffee table that God is not looking for flash and dash. He's looking for plodders. Staying in the game was Iron Mike.

I sat at the kitchen table, considering what to do now. I remembered the Missoula urologist who counseled Mike. He told Mike that if his PSA started to elevate, we were to look for a medical oncologist in Minneapolis specializing in treating prostate cancer.

"These physicians have better therapies for addressing advanced prostate cancer," he had said.

Our exhilaration from thinking Mike could be off his medication plummeted to a despairing concern that we had made a mistake. Undaunted, I took the Missoula urologist's suggestion and dove into finding the best specialists in Minneapolis for treating prostate cancer. Contacting my first choice, I soon learned we had to apply, sending all the records from Mayo Clinic. *What are this doctor's acceptance criteria? Will Mike's case qualify? What could be more challenging than this newly awakened metastatic cancer?* To me, the tumor marker ticking up meant the cancer was growing somewhere in his body. We needed action.

Finally, we heard the news we wanted to hear. Our chosen oncologist had accepted Mike as a patient. He was a specialist who garnered high ratings as one of the best cancer oncologists in our area. Considering these recent changes, I wondered about the road ahead for us. Giving it all up to God, I prayed, "God, here we are again. We don't know the road ahead, but You lead us."

As I set up an appointment with our new specialist, my thoughts tumbled to questions. *What about healing? Is the arm of the Lord too short? How shall we pray now?* Our lives seemed like spilled milk flowing down the table legs. Could it be contained again the way it had been before?

STRATEGY | *JUNE 2013*

Traveling downtown to meet Mike's new oncologist, we waited in a tiny consultation room on the second floor. To break the stress, Mike entertained himself with one of the hand puzzles on the windowsill while I flipped through a joke book. Finally, Mike queried, "Do you think he will have a better plan to keep the PSA down?"

"Well, he certainly has different training with different therapies."

I hoped someone had a better plan. A nurse came into our small consultation room and explained she would be our nurse hereafter with our doctor. After taking a history and checking vital signs, she said the doctor would see Mike. On her way out, she hinted that the doctor might interject humor. I liked that thought. *This serious cancer business has sharp edges.*

As the oncologist entered our consultation room, he immediately enlivened the place with his smile and upbeat, casual manner, interjecting several quips to put Mike at ease. Mike was cautious at first, but the doctor's disarming charm, warmth, and wit made Mike quickly relax. The oncologist wanted to get to know Mike, what he liked to do, and how long we had been married. I saw the immediate connection between these two, especially in humor. The uneasiness I knew Mike felt on the way to this clinic vanished entirely.

The oncologist's apparent clarity of direction in managing Mike's case engendered our confidence at once. At the same time, Mike's recent negative news hung in our minds. The oncologist explained he had plans to keep the cancer in check. But, first, he wanted Mike to stay on the original drug. Mike was visibly disheartened. But the doctor seemed to have a strategy and encouraged Mike to listen.

The doctor elucidated a management plan utterly different from our current one. Instead of killing the cancer, his approach would be to keep the disease at bay. Then, explaining a new therapy he had in mind, he took a piece of paper and drew a schematic of the pathway of how the original drug worked. Then on top of that, he drew a different way the new drug would work. I liked the visuals.

Mike soon understood the oncologist wanted him to be on both drugs simultaneously.

"Why do I have to stay on the original drug? I don't want those side effects."

"The cancer mutated," the oncologist explained. "Some cells are different now, while other cells remain the same. The original drug fights those cells that have not changed, while the new drug will block the pathway of changed cells."

My question was, "How does cancer happen in the first place?"

"As cells age, the natural life cycle is that they should die at some point. However, cancer cells don't want to die. These cells try to prolong their lives by extending into other locations in the body."

This cancer changes its identity; it morphs into something different to escape the battle! How insidious!

MORE GEAR | *SPRING 2014*

With more visits to this new doctor, we felt at least someone was in control. That someone was not only the new doctor, but we had to let God be in charge. We were not running the ship. We felt encouraged about the direction ahead. Things seemed under control with Mike's PSA staying low.

Before the next checkup, Mike wanted to purchase a new chainsaw. He had three chainsaws in Montana but also needed one in Minneapolis. His goal was clearing small trees and brush beginning to obscure our marsh view. Deciding he also required the accompanying gear, we traveled across town to an equipment store, complete with every type of Stihl outdoor machine. *More gear, duplicating everything we already have in*

Montana—chainsaw, protective eyewear, specially lined pants, jacket, gloves, and helmet.

We ended that gear-buying day at the oncology clinic for Mike's next appointment. Sitting in the small examination room, Mike's oncologist entered and smiled as he shook Mike's hand. The day before, we were at this same clinic when they had drawn Mike's blood for testing.

"How are things going, Mike? Did you run today?" The oncologist wanted to understand how Mike was feeling.

Mike was feeling more at ease with every visit with this doctor. Knowing the doctor could be humorous, Mike relaxed. Their quick interchange of comments and banter became a style Mike loved. Mike and I also liked the doctor's direct way of telling things as they were. We needed to understand how Mike was doing and appreciated the doctor's openness and honesty.

After the initial pleasantries, the oncologist informed Mike that his blood marker was increasing. With that, our alarm ratcheted up. But I saw the oncologist was eager to explain his next plan. "Your surgery at Mayo removed your original tumor and cancerous lymph nodes. Any increase now of tumor marker signals new growth somewhere in your body. We need to locate where this is," he summarized. He wanted Mike to undergo a series of tests and scans to define the cause of this finding. Mike was on board. Charge ahead!

In a few days, we were back to hear the results of the scans. The doctor said Mike needed radiation for a small nodule of disease in his groin. "This radiation," he said, "will precisely target that nodule, and then we'll see you in three months."

Mike's spirits were high as he started radiation treatments. As he completed the series, his radiation oncologist said he weathered the procedures better than most, probably due to his otherwise excellent physical health and conditioning. After one radiation visit, Mike wanted to stop downtown at the Filson clothing store to see the new season's offerings. His collection of clothes, shoes, and outdoor wear filled closets at our Minnesota home and in Montana. He was the best-dressed man I knew. I sometimes felt shabby next to him because I hated to shop. I let Mike be Mike that day. Lovable Mike. It was his escape.

STEPWISE | *SUMMER 2014*

With positive results from the radiation treatments, we relaxed to enjoy that summer at our Minneapolis home. Mike liked to maintain our lawn, keeping it in immaculate shape, the envy of the neighborhood. He had fun zipping around the yard in twenty minutes with the zero-turn riding mower he'd purchased the previous year. When we bought our house, Mike had a sprinkler system installed, so the yard would remain verdant even when we were in Montana. My job included trimming the bushes and maintaining the flower beds, the latter mostly populated with perennials, including irises from my grandmother's garden I'd planted several years before she passed. Elated that my Jackmanii clematis was now in full bloom, I recalled some years I missed my grandmother's irises blooming altogether due to our vagabond lifestyle.

As I walked about our lawn inspecting flowers and plants, I thought about how I wanted God to give the doctor wisdom for the right strategy to combat Mike's cancer. I thought back over Mike's checkup visits. When the results were positive, the oncologist wanted Mike to stay the course. We loved his enthusiasm and positive outlook. I loved that Mike relied on the oncologist and looked forward to his visits with him. I trusted the doctor to determine the next steps. Yet, I still wanted God as our true Director and continued to plead for His wisdom to cover the oncologist in his decisions.

Is it wrong to have faith that the cancer would be thwarted? I knew not everyone who prayed that prayer got healed. We didn't want to give up on praying for healing. I wanted the Lord to contend with those who contended with us, to fight against those who were fighting with us. I trusted the Lord would miraculously heal Mike, and we would have a great story to tell everyone. This story would be about how the great I AM worked in Mike's life.

God was the One who could keep our souls quiet through these ups and downs. As I gave this playbook into God's hand, I knew the outcome would play out exactly as He planned. So I bowed to the Lord Almighty again.

You are in charge. I know You are Sovereign. No plan of Yours can be thwarted.

But I am not ready for Mike to go to heaven just yet.

PLODDING | *NOVEMBER 2014*

We faced another appointment on a gray day in Minneapolis, where the clouds shrouded the earth in dreary sameness. Yet, not knowing what this day's results would be, we maintained our spirits despite the overcast surroundings. As we entered the muted-toned waiting room of our clinic, Mike chatted with the receptionist as I sat wondering why waiting rooms never had upbeat color schemes or colors that would inspire someone to get up and dance.

I'M GOING TO RUN UNTIL I'M DONE

Escorting us into a tiny exam room, the nurse took Mike's vital signs and asked Mike how he was doing. She revealed nothing about Mike's PSA test results and said the doctor would be right in.

"Mike, your numbers are up," the doctor said as he entered the room. Then, he told Mike about a different drug he wanted to try. I could see how deflated Mike was. Yet the doctor remained optimistic, and before we left the clinic, he prescribed the next therapy. *Here we go again.*

We went home, and as usual, Mike announced he was going on a run. Before he walked out the door, he looked back at me and declared, "It's spread, but I'm not dead."

I saw the hope he maintained. It reminded me I should keep that hope as well. He left me sitting in my chair, asking God, "What is Your will here, Lord? What if our prayers are incongruous with Your will? What if we are deluding ourselves? What if healing never comes for Mike? How should I think about this?"

I reminded myself God is only good. Bad things do not come from Him. I knew from the Word that we live in this fallen world, its brokenness everywhere with sickness, disease, and evil. It began back in the Garden days. Before the fall of humankind, the created world was perfect. Someday, I thought, we would be in a perfect environment in heaven. Eternity past and eternity future were like bookends sandwiching humanity's time on earth. Although the middle chapter might seem the best or only part to some people, our senses cannot fully perceive the best is yet to come. In this middle part, we have the Perfect One to go with us through our trials and heartbreaks.

I also knew I did not have the entire picture of what was

happening, nor did I truly want the whole movie. I had to be satisfied that God was Sovereign. He was the One in control, not me. Even though these cancer vignettes playing out in our lives did not look so good, I needed to surrender to let Him be God. He *"works all things according to the counsel of His will"* (Ephesians 1:11, NKJV).

Lord, this is hard, I prayed. Please help us through all of this. With You, I want to *"be strong in the Lord and in the power of His might"* (Ephesians 6:10, NKJV).

GETAWAY | *NOVEMBER 2014*

After hearing the news Mike's PSA was increasing, we flew to Montana. The two-and-a-half-hour plane trip left us with enough energy for the rest of the day. On that cold day, I built a fire in our cabin fireplace. The dancing flames licked the larch logs I had loaded. The towering stone fireplace nearly reached the twenty-five-foot wood beam-lined cathedral ceiling. Although the side walls were mainly windows overlooking the front forest and the back meadow, the great room remained dim that day. Glancing at the substantial horizontal beams supporting the pitched roof, I reviewed the happenings of the last few months. New drugs and radiation took a toll on Mike, but he still had the resilience and perseverance to keep his exercise routine. I could see he was trying to stay strong. Could we possibly plan another big trip between his three-month intervals of doctor visits? I had ideas.

In the previous two years, I had ventured into discovering my ancestors on the Ancestry online site. I needed a diversion from the string of negative doctor results. I knew my lineage on my mother's side but lacked information on my father's side.

My father, an only child, died when I was very young. With no first cousins, I lacked much knowledge of his family.

I became acquainted with a third cousin from Illinois on the Ancestry website. She and I talked of a trip to Wales one day, where my great-grandfather and my cousin's great-grandmother were born. I had researched my father's side of the family for two years. My great-grandfather wrote letters back to his relatives in Wales after he immigrated to the United States in 1853. In those letters, I learned the names of people and farms where his siblings lived in Wales. Those clues, plus searching an Ancestry site, revealed a genealogy with our family surname and the same first names as my great-grandfather's children. I sent a message to the owner of that Ancestry site, querying if we may be related, but received no response.

After a year and a half, I finally received a reply from that Ancestry site. The responding person connected me with a woman named Jean Davies, who descended from that family. Unfortunately, she disclosed little about my connection to her ancestors but invited me to visit if I ever came to Wales.

I also discovered a published book containing the history of a Welsh family with my surname from my online research. It detailed the same farm names as in my great-grandfather's letters. So, procuring that book and scouring its clues, I put two and two together, thinking this family could be relatives.

My Illinois cousin and I seriously began to consider a trip to Wales. Would Mike have the stamina for such a trip? "We could squeeze it in between doctor visits," I told him. He did not say no, so I jumped into planning the trip. My sister also wanted to go, so I booked the trip for the following summer, hoping all would be well for Mike to go. I purposely selected the time for the trip around the British Open Golf Tournament, just in case Mike felt well enough to take it in. That was the plan.

DESIGN | *SUMMER 2015*

Mike could help us navigate on this trip, I thought. With his next check-up not until September, we had the break we needed to squeeze in the trip to Wales. Landing outside Cardiff, a stiff breeze blew off the ocean as we piled our suitcases into the rental car we booked. Driving on the wrong side of the road took some brain adjustment. With all the connecting circles and spider-webbed roads, it took all our effort to read the signs and maps to arrive at the meeting with our potential newfound relative. We were full of expectations.

We navigated to Jean Davies' village, about twenty miles from the airport. Meeting us outside her tidy, white-framed home, Jean smiled and welcomed us. I could hardly contain myself. Taking us inside, Jean introduced us to her first cousin, Janet, and Janet's husband, then ushered us into her reception room. Immediately they wanted to know about our flight and driving on their road system. After these opening pleasantries, Jean, our hostess, served tea with Bara Brith, a traditional Welsh bread baked with currents soaked in tea, citrus, and spices. Janet, her cousin, introduced us to Welsh cakes covered in powdered sugar, another Welsh favorite. All the while, I am exploding inside, wondering, *are you our relatives?*

We began the story of our great-grandparents emigrating from Wales, my great-grandmother dying of cholera on the ship, and the settlement of our widowed great-grandfather and his ten children in the Midwest. Then, quietly, Jean exited the room and came back in, unrolling a huge genealogy chart that included my great-grandfather's family.

"Finally!" I exclaimed jubilantly. I could barely contain myself! Jean and Janet were third cousins descending from the same forefathers and on the same farm. Until that moment, I had doubted whether this trip would uncover anything about my father's ancestry.

Elated by that discovery, we left our new cousin's home to find the farm mentioned in my great-grandfather's letters. Driving through narrow, overgrown hedged roads, winding up a hill, we came to a gate with the sign Llechartfach, the farm in my great-grandfather's letters. The gate was closed.

We looked at each other, our minds racing about our next move, knowing we would never come this way again.

"Should we open it?" Abandoning our hesitation, one of us pushed the gate open and swung it to the side. We slowly drove the long lane to the top of the hill to the house and farm buildings nestled there. Feeling like we trespassed, I hoped someone was home.

I had researched this farm online a year earlier and found the present owner's name. I had sent him a letter explaining this could be the farm where my ancestors lived, and if we made a trip to Wales, could we visit? But unfortunately, I never received a reply.

A dark-haired man dressed in his work clothes came out of an old white-plastered stone house to meet us. I could tell he was questioning who we were and why we were there. I introduced ourselves and explained this farm may be the one written in my great-grandfather's letters and may have been their ancestral homestead and birthplace.

"Did you receive the letter I wrote, maybe more than a year

ago? My great-grandfather mentioned Llechartfach farm in his letters. He visited that farm when he returned to Wales in the early 1870s."

"Yes, your letter is still in my diary. I am sorry I did not respond at that time. My mother, who also lived here, was very ill then. She passed two months ago. I just never got around to responding."

"We are so sorry about your mother," I offered, realizing then that extenuating circumstances in everyone's lives constrain us from appropriately responding when we should.

"Thank you. I can show you the place now. This is the original house, over three hundred years old and occupied all this time. I live here now. As you can see, this home features the original stone construction."

We toured the inside with low wood-beamed ceilings and white plastered stone walls. The owner showed us the stone staircase leading to two upstairs bedrooms. Outside he took us to a field with a view that took our breath away. From that hilltop, the ocean at Swansea Bay was the backdrop in the far distance for the rolling green pastures dotted with sheep. This idyllic scene was like a picture postcard of the Welsh landscape; green stone-fenced fields with the shimmering blue ocean in the background.

With his tour, my history holes began filling in. As we departed and thanked the present owner, he directed us a mile down the road to visit Gellionen Chapel, where he said some of our ancestors were probably buried. *More discovery!*

A profound sense of connectedness with my father, his family, and their history overwhelmed me. He would love to know we visited his ancestral home. Our visit to Llechartfach, with its surrounding beauty and vistas, cemented a sense of place within me, a sense of belonging. My soul felt full. I wanted to linger and relish the moments.

That day a part of me stayed on that hill.

Full of excitement with the discoveries of this trip, I knew the rest of the journey would be easier for Mike. He needed to rest.

We had previously booked the remainder of the trip in Scotland because my Illinois cousin's paternal ancestors were Scottish. After arriving in Edinburgh on Saturday, we checked into our downtown hotel and took time to relax in the late afternoon sun.

The following morning, Mike and I walked around the city center near our hotel. In front of us was the Balmoral Hotel.

"Let's look inside." He wanted to take in the interior of this grand hotel with its auspicious name. Across the lobby, he saw a table displaying a British Open Golf Tournament sign. Mike bee-lined to that table with two ladies sitting behind it.

"How far is the tournament from here?"

"Just a half-hour train ride to St. Andrews. Would you like tickets for the weather-delayed final day tomorrow? Many attendees have international flights home today, and will not be attending the final round, so we have inexpensive tickets for the Monday conclusion."

A big smile came over Mike's face. "Would I?" He exclaimed. "How much are the tickets?"

The lady explained that they were offering tickets at a considerable discount because they wanted a large crowd for the last day on Monday.

"How would we get there?"

"The train is just outside this hotel under the street. You would be there in a half-hour."

"And the cost of the train?"

"About fifteen pounds."

Mike looked at me with excitement in his eyes. I could see he was weighing this as a chance of a lifetime. He never dreamed he would have this opportunity.

She said a bus would be at the train station in St. Andrews, shuttling attendees to the Old Course for the tournament.

The following day after a hearty Scottish breakfast of bacon and eggs at our hotel, we walked a half block to board the train to St. Andrews. A bus picked us up at St. Andrews and carried us to the Old Course. I knew Mike would like to walk around the course and see the play at different holes. However, we both knew he did not have the energy. So, we positioned ourselves in the stands alongside the 18th hole with a view of the Swilcan Bridge. There we watched as groups came in, one by one.

Mike became a chatterbox the whole time about the players, their shots, and their scores. He was in his element. I was someplace else. *This entire trip was designed for discovering my family roots, and we did that! But God had something more. Here we were, sitting at the Old Course at St. Andrew's. Not in his lifetime or in his condition would Mike imagine he would attend the British Open. And on this day, when an Iowan won the tournament!*

MONTANA LIFE | *SEPTEMBER 2015*

Buoyed by our British Isles adventure, we came home to another check-up for Mike. His PSA test results were not good, so the oncologist decided on a new drug. I could see Mike's despondency about his status but also his resignation to the doctor's care and plan. The new drug was an oral one, so after procuring it, we flew to Montana, our place for quiet and reflection. Mike's childhood dream and love for the mountains led him to search for this place, a retreat that was a statement about him. It was his idea of paradise. Mike loved his Montana home, outfitted with a buffalo head-mount on the tall stone fireplace, artisan pieces, and western paintings. When alpenglow graced Van's Peak and Swan Peak in the evening, he loved to sit on the deck, basking in its golden brilliance.

Inside the house, we arrayed pictures of the animals that had visited our property over our time there. Recently, a taffy-colored grizzly made itself evident on our property. Scat was everywhere. That animal left other clues, too. Bite marks in the garden hose converted it into a sprinkler. We found teeth marks in the deck wood, demolished security signs, and a dented wheelbarrow. This bear returned later the same evening, so we called the DNR. They brought a bear trap the size of a pickup truck, outfitted with cameras and baited with a hind quarter of deer. Thank God, this bear moved on.

Another time we stayed indoors on a drizzly day when a mountain lion meandered up to our deck and peered into our closed sliding glass doors. This lion looked in at us as if we were in a cage. Like death approaching our door, my heart raced at this juxtaposition. We assumed the glass reflected the lion's image like a mirror. Later we learned of a lion having kittens on the deck of a neighbor's home a mile away while she was absent for the winter. Perhaps our lion was accustomed to decks.

CELEBRATION | *JANUARY 2016*

Mike ran on the Luce Line Trail in good weather, but not on snowy days. Instead, Mike listened to music with earphones while running on his treadmill. He determined to get his run in before we went to another clinic appointment. *Another run to be recorded in his logbook.* Each new therapy left him listless, yet he continued to run. Running was his therapy, and this escape kept him in the game. I also knew he could not run without music. Music filled our living spaces: CDs in our home, XM in the cars, and at our Montana home. You name it; his music was playing everywhere. He required music. When I found the book, *Your Brain on Music*, I bought it to understand this fix. I imagined music transported his brain to another place.

We jumped in the car to drive to the oncologist's suburban clinic just ten minutes away. As we backed out of the driveway, Mike tuned the radio to XM for some upbeat music. We loved not having to go to our oncologist's downtown clinic on this inclement day. At this clinic, Mike began to know each nurse. I wondered if they saw Mike as I did, a person you just wanted to hug.

Over the last year, Mike's oncologist had tried several cancer drugs to combat Mike's reappearing cancer, most without success. At this clinic visit, the nurse ushered us into one of the small examination rooms. After checking vital signs and asking the usual questions, she announced that Mike's PSA had declined substantially. When the doctor entered the room, Mike sang The Rascals' "Good Lovin'" song.

"Doctor, Doctor, Mr. M.D., Can you tell me what's ailing me?"

The doctor smiled and informed us that tune was his ringtone to other doctors. This levity opened the conversation about how Mike was doing. Was he running? How was he feeling?

This day was a happy one. The nurse returned with a graphed picture of the last three months' results. Textbook-perfect, this chemotherapy had worked.

Finally, we had a winning strategy. We went home elated, thinking *Mike will now have a stable period*. Mike and I talked about the bloodwork results and how excited the doctor was about the graph showing a considerable drop in tumor marker. Encouraged and relieved, we were thankful that we finally had a working plan.

A YEAR | *JUNE 2016*

Early one morning, as I sat on our porch finishing my second cup of coffee, I reflected on Mike's condition. He was still running, albeit at a much slower pace. On the Luce Line Trail, Mike would turn off his music and stop to talk when he saw friends and acquaintances. I was sure he wanted some sympathy along the way for his challenging situation. Most people probably found it unbelievable Mike still had any energy to exercise. But they could see his resolution to continue by how slowly he ran. I, too, pitied him with hot flashes, fatigue, and weight gain from the original drug, exacerbated by the side effects of each added drug.

I knew God was using these encounters for His purposes. Mike was fighting the battle of his life. He trusted God, and the people he met listened as he told them that God was there in the battle. As Mike told me about these encounters, I prayed for each person that Mike's words about God would be sticky

—that the words would stay in their minds—causing them to honestly consider God.

We were still basking in the good results from the previous visit as we returned to the clinic for Mike's next check-up. After the nurse took Mike's history and vitals, we waited a few moments for the doctor to enter the room. In the past, we had learned if Mike's results were good, the nurse revealed the results. If the results were not good, the doctor brought the news. It suddenly dawned on me that the nurse had not told Mike his results this time. *Was negative news impending?* As I processed what this could mean, the doctor entered the room, greeted us, and asked Mike how he was doing. Mike went down a list of things that were not right but said he was still running.

"Mike, your PSA is up again." *How could the excellent news of a few months ago go down the drain so fast? Doesn't anything last?*

The oncologist took his chair before his computer and retrieved Mike's report on his screen. And leaning forward to put his hand on Mike's knee, he said, "Mike, you have a year to live." And after a pause, "I wish I had better news."

"Years?" Mike shot back, trying to negotiate for more time. I knew Mike was the consummate negotiator, and he would give all he had to get a better forecast.

But the doctor repeated those exact words, "You have a year to live."

Oh, no, can this be?

After this exchange, the doctor seemed to be having a conversation with himself about how our culture elevates life so high that death is never considered; how people do not want to think about death as part of life. After that, he

I'M GOING TO RUN UNTIL I'M DONE

continued his conversation with himself—it is a natural sequence, a part of life to be accepted.

Then the oncologist asked, "Mike, where do you want to die?"

Mike quickly answered, "At home."

This rapid-fire volley hit me, leaving their exchange echoing in my brain, with neon lights flashing A Year! I could not believe we were at this point. *What about our summer plans for having family visit us in Montana? What is the plan ahead?*

Then the doctor offered, "If you need anything, anything at all, you can call the clinic." Then he wrote his cell phone number on a paper from his desk and gave it to Mike. Before that moment, I had not considered that giving negative news to patients might also be hard on doctors.

Not prepared for any of this, I was nowhere near considering this timeframe for Mike. *Are we really at this point?* I had never gotten that far in my thinking, not even close. In my mind, I thought this stage of chemo and radiation would go on and on, never considering an endpoint. Was I blind to blank that out? Broaching this subject was unthinkable before. Now, it stared me in the face. Mike wanted to die at our home.

Back home, my mind raced. *What about all Your promises, Lord? Your miracles? Where are You now? Don't leave us stranded. Help us!* We hightailed for the porch, our talking place. But we were silent. *How do things turn south overnight?* I wanted to know how we got to this juncture so fast without warning. I knew oncologists needed to understand the patient's wishes early in the game and document those directions in their clinic notes. Then, when the time came, they knew which way to go. *But this is heavy news!* I was sure Mike also was shocked at the doctor's announcement, but I saw him let these words evaporate so he could carry on. Finally, after a few minutes, he said, "I'm going running."

As Mike left me sitting there to ponder this new prognosis and this place of dying twist thrown into the mix, I was amazed at how little this news seemed to affect him, yet I knew inside Mike was crying.

I agonized over this awful news and all this talk about dying, so weighty, closing in on us, like a heavy iron door slowly shutting, allowing no way to escape. I broke down. *Lord, help us through this. Help me through this.*

Trying to regain some semblance of what to do next, I searched through my card verses. I wanted the one that said, *"Don't be afraid, for I have called you by name; you are mine. When you go through deep waters and great trouble, I will be with you. When you go through rivers of difficulty, you will not drown! When you walk through the fire of oppression, you will not be burned up—the flames will not consume you. For I am the Lord, your God, your Savior"* (Isaiah 43:1-3 NIV).

After that terrible news, we decided to bolt to Montana. I took that verse and other verses along with us. We both needed time to reflect on those words and the doctor's words. We needed breathing space to reflect on where we were now.

Arriving at our Montana home, I slumped into my deck chair. Majestic Van's Peak framed the eighty-foot Douglas fir in the back corner of our property. My world was falling in on me. I wanted time to think and talk with God. My questions spilled out as tears flowed down my cheeks. Overwhelmed by the thought that Mike's end was near, I silently asked God, "Are You working everything out for good?" I wanted to say to Him, "I don't know Your plan for Mike, for us, but this does not look good."

I knew I had to let go of my always-trying-to-be-in-control mode. I knew I was not calling the shots; God was. He was in charge. God knew this was going to happen. *Help, Lord. Only You know the way ahead of us.*

REFLECTION

The following day as I sat on a deck chair, I watched two dragonflies circling the open meadow, landing on the long, unmown grass. Surrounded by the glorious Swan Valley, I contemplated that every day at this Montana home felt like another day in paradise. Each day was a copycat of the previous day. Each night the temperature dropped to the low 40s as the cold air from the Mission Mountains and the Swan peaks settled into our valley. It made for great sleeping; wool blankets required.

The sun's warmth and the serenity of the scene overwhelmed me. Even in our calamity, God was trying to show me His glory, calmness, and peace. After a late bacon and eggs breakfast, Mike ambled toward the garage. He wanted me to follow him. Weary from the work he tried the day before of limbing a log and helping burn a slash pile, he realized he could no longer do all the outdoor work he used to do. I felt sad as I watched him climb on the ATV, barely managing to lift his leg over the seat. Sapped of energy, I could tell he was not happy about his status, but he maintained a determination to get things done. Driving the ATV out of the way, he started the riding mower. Motioning me to his side, he wanted *me* to learn how to use the riding mower to clip the grassy area around the house. I grasped he was signaling about the future without him, something I did not want to consider.

Before this time, Mike's responsibilities included the outside work and machinery (boy toys). Not familiar with his riding mower, I required a bit of training. After reviewing the gears and how to start the mower, I hoped I could master the machine. Mike sat on the deck, directing me as I circled, cutting the area behind the house, around the fire pit, and out as far as the slash pile.

As I mowed, I replayed a conversation Mike and I had early in our marriage about trusting the God of the Bible. At that time, Mike had queried whether we could trust God at His Word. One of Mike's questions then concerned Jesus. Was He the Messiah, or had He coincidentally fulfilled many Old Testament prophecies? I told Mike then that somewhere, I had read how someone calculated the probability of Jesus fulfilling Old Testament prophecies about the Messiah. If one chose just eight of the 300+ Old Testament prophecies about Jesus and calculated the statistical probability of the likelihood of this happening by chance alone, it would be highly improbable. And if Jesus fulfilled all the 300+ prophecies of the Old Testament, how many times more unlikely would that be?[1]

That conversation continued in my mind. I remembered relaying what I read about the British mathematician, astronomer, and astrobiologist Chandra Wickramasinghe. He had calculated the statistical probability of just one of the one-thousand human cell enzymes formed by chance alone. He calculated this to be 1 times 10 to the 40,000th power.[2]

"Do you know what that means?" I asked Mike.

"What?"

"Well, one multiplied by 10 to the 3rd power would mean there is one chance in a thousand that something would happen. One in a million is 10 to the 6th power. One multiplied by ten to the 40,000th power would mean one with 40,000 zeros behind the number 1—an infinitesimally minuscule probability of this happening by chance alone."

Wickramasinghe wrote a rebuttal to the claim that neo-Darwinian evolution was a proven fact. His calculation about one single human enzyme coming into being by chance alone was, as he wrote, a "really vast improbability . . . that posed a serious dilemma for the whole of evolutionary science." Thus, he concluded, "Life could not be an accident, not just on the Earth, but anywhere, anywhere at all in the Universe."

"This would be improbable at the highest level," I said to Mike. "To have just one enzyme come into being simultaneous with the thousands of other cell enzymes also coming into being. The probability of this happening by chance alone is unexplainable without an Intelligent Designer, that being God."

At that time, our conversation turned to other reasons the universe was not a chance happening. I relayed to Mike that our planet in our galaxy appears exquisitely placed to be inhabitable by life. Any deviation from this placement by a minute degree would not allow life. This exact placement pointed to fine-tuning by a Master Fine Tuner. "It's like a sweet-spot set-up, in a very narrow window of circumstances, that we live. And, amazingly, it is all there for our discovery. The best fit for the evidence is a worldview with God as Creator."

Mike followed with, "The whole Bible all hangs together."

"And it's not contradictory, and it all points to the coming of the Messiah—Jesus." I described the unity of the Bible to him—sixty-six books by forty authors written over several thousand years, all pointing to the Messiah. And these writings are not contradictory to archeology, history, or science. On the contrary, the more we uncover or discover, the more evidence supports the Scriptures. The Bible has significantly influenced the world and survives despite attempts to wipe it out. And would the disciples have given their lives for someone who was a fake or a fraud? The most telling evidence," I said, "is how people's lives are radically changed. Your best evidence is your own life and how your life changed when you let Jesus be Lord. My personal best proof is the overwhelming peace and assurance I have. We can intellectually see how this worldview, with God as Creator, makes the best sense of any worldview. It is the Holy Spirit who assures us this is all true."

I remember Mike had listened intently but stayed silent. I saw he thought about what he read in the Bible, all those promises God made to believers, and the assurance he felt. I could see the whole thing made sense to him more than any other explanation. *God is for real. He is overall; He created all. Here we are, walking through our ordeal. All I need is to let Him be God. He knows the end from the beginning.*

As I finished mowing, I carefully backed the mower into the crowded garage, housing all Mike's "toys."

AGAIN | *AUGUST 2016*

With all the wildlife and beautiful scenery in Montana, sometimes we stayed for months between doctor visits and chemotherapy. But it was time for another clinic visit. So back at home, as we prepared for that visit, I resigned myself to what we might hear. This time the doctor informed Mike the latest scans showed tumor growth in two new areas. He wanted to do radiation to zap those spots. Mike and I agreed with his plan. *What else can we do?* So for the next fifteen days, we traveled to the downtown hospital for a fifteen-minute radiation procedure.

After completing that radiation series, Mike came to our porch and uttered in the lingo of the 1840s mountain men, "They kilt me, but I still lived." He had survived the radiation well, with no untoward effects, but I saw the change in him. After that, I kept my feelings to myself, a task I could do well. Raised in a primarily Mennonite community, where little children hovered behind their parents, letting the others do the talking, I remember rarely opening my mouth.

I pondered the last couple of years as Mike trekked through several different chemotherapies and radiation series. When the tumor marker ticked up, the oncologist had a new strategy. It seemed the oncologist had many tricks in his bag. He never seemed to run out of ideas for the next steps. The efficacy of each determined what was next. We were waiting on the hand of God for every outcome. I remembered the verse in Psalm 27:14, *"Wait on the Lord; Be of good courage, And He shall strengthen your heart; Wait, I say, on the Lord!"* (NKJV). I prayed, "Waiting is hard, Lord, when results are bad, but I trust You to keep us when we cannot keep ourselves."

During these days, I found it hard to watch Mike barely running. Some people walked faster than he ran. Refusing to give up, even in his weakened condition, when he became too weak to finish his run, he would stop altogether and sit on a curb until someone stopped and drove him home. I started driving to his halfway point to bring him a drink of ice water and cheer him on. I knew he would not give up running.

I'll never forget when Mike told his oncologist during one clinic visit, "I am going to run until I'm done."

"You are not done yet," the doctor declared. That was the endorsement Mike wanted to hear. *Hallelujah, we have time left!*

The oncologist had a sequence of chemotherapies he was trying, perhaps determined by clinical trials. We knew at least one of them gave a temporary halting of the cancer in the past. Others had failed miserably.

During this time, Mike began referring to himself as "Chemo Sabe." Accompanying each round of chemotherapy was a long list of after-effects: the total sick feeling that Mike could not put into words, energy depletion, fluid retention, foggy chemo-brain, thinning skin, and the appearance of bruises. Along with these chemotherapies came drug-related deleterious effects of bone density loss and compromised immune system. The doctor then ordered other drugs to combat these depletions and protect his immune system.

Around this time, Mikey's right leg became fluid-filled, which the oncologist said was due to blockage of the lymph system from previous radiation treatments. He referred Mike to a physical medicine specialist for something called lymphedema. As we waited for that doctor to enter the small examination room, Mike immediately turned to a human skeleton hanging from a metal stand next to the doctor's chair. Mike jumped up and put the skeleton's dangling right arm around his neck. Taking a quick picture with my iPhone, we both smiled at Mike's opportunity to interject a little levity into his ongoing cancer saga. He quickly resumed his chair beside the doctor's desk.

When the doctor entered, she opened his file on her computer to review the reason for this appointment. I could not help but share Mike's picture with her, making her smile. This physical medicine doctor had seen other cancer patients with Mike's present problem. Some previous treatment, perhaps radiation, was now blocking lymph flow in that leg back to his body core. To control the incoming fluid into the leg, she prescribed a tight stocking for his whole leg.

Undaunted by this new encumbrance, Mike determined to run, even with this tight stocking. The skin-colored stocking did not match the tone of his other leg. After one run, Mike told me another runner approached him from behind and asked, "Is that a prosthetic leg?" Opportunity! Mike launched into his spiel about his cancer story.

Back at home, I sat on our porch, deep in thought. *How will this play out? Will my Mikey be dead in a year?*

I wanted to encourage Mike, but really, I was the one who needed encouragement. God knew this trail we were on. He knew the end from the beginning; our job was to stay close to Him. Our times were in His hand.

A song from my childhood came to mind.

> God leads His dear children along
> Some through the waters,
> Some through the flood,
> Some through the fire,
> But all through the blood.
> Some through great sorrow,
> But God gives a song,
> In the night season and all the day long.
> ("God Leads Us Along" by G. A. Young)

I realized we were walking across this chemotherapy valley, yet I knew God promised to be right there beside us. That reminded me of my mother's old, framed picture, now hanging in a guest bedroom. The background depicted a tremendous storm with lightning piercing the black sky. Two young children are crossing a rickety bridge over a rushing stream. Over them and protecting them is this tall, glorious angel. *That's Mike and me crossing this cancer chasm. We are under God's care and keeping. He gives His angels charge over us.*

When I relayed my thoughts about this picture to Mike, he asked, "Will you be able to carry on after I am gone?"

I assured him I would, an automatic response even though I had not allowed my brain to entertain what it would be like to live without him. I just wanted us both to persevere in this fight. With God's help, this rickety bridge where we were contending with cancer was our stand in faith. All I knew was we needed His leading.

I wanted God to lead the way. I wanted Him to be our Pilot. I thought back to a time at work when I had an appointment to see a physician in a different state. I had flown overnight and rented a car to travel from my hotel to the hospital, where I would meet our company representative and this physician. With driving instructions, I allowed enough time to get to the hospital before the meeting began. Unfortunately, I got lost because I took a wrong turn, circling back to the same place three times. Knowing this university hospital would be huge, I scanned the horizon, thinking I should see it. Not seeing any tall buildings and not knowing what road to take, I audibly prayed, "Lord, You're going to have to get me there." Just then, a shiny, black, vintage pick-up truck swerved close in front of me. His license plate read: God is My Pilot.

God, I guess I am supposed to follow that truck. So as the truck turned the corner, I followed. Within a couple of minutes, I arrived at the hospital just in time for my meeting.

SCENE | *SEPTEMBER 2016*

After we waded through all of Mike's appointments, we again fled to Montana, where we soaked in the late morning sun on our Montana deck. In the distance, I heard a squirrel scolding and, even farther away, several ravens squawking back and forth. We had invaded their territory. Too bad. We just wanted to sit and relax.

A pair of gray jays swooped into our clearing. Their soft, fluid notes, high in the trees, gave a sublime layer to our morning. I pondered the short scope of this life. I knew, at some point, I would have a conversation that might help Mike think about the afterlife. Until this point, I detected he was not ready to talk about dying. But he knew from his Bible reading that we go immediately to be with Jesus the second we die.

I thought we were at a different juncture now, and he might be more amenable to discussing what comes next, even though I knew him to be a live-in-the-moment person. I tested the waters. "I wonder what my mother is doing in heaven right now. And Brad?" My mother had been in heaven for years, my brother for decades. Just thinking about their life there now encouraged me.

"What do you think heaven will be like?" Mike queried. I got up from my sunny deck chair and went into the house to retrieve some Scripture verses I'd brought along on this trip. I had waited a long time for this conversation.

Coming back to my deck chair, I saw that he was open to thinking about this. "The most welcoming Presence in heaven will be Jesus. In heaven, His love will envelop us, enfold us, and hold us," I looked at him, and seeing he was intently listening, I continued, "We will not need faith there because our faith will have become sight. Remember what you wrote on that card you placed on the porch table at home about faith?"

"No, I don't remember." I could tell he wanted to hear more.

"You wrote that faith is the confident assurance that what we hope for is going to happen. It is the evidence of things we cannot see."

I went on to describe how I imagined heaven. "All of our hopes will be made real. We will experience His fullness and our wholeness; we will be thrilled beyond imagination, wholly satisfied, safe, and secure. In His Presence, we will see His face. We will see all this with our eyes and our spirit. We will be more alive than we ever knew we could be. We will be delighted beyond our wildest imagination. And I think we will be astounded by God explaining the hidden treasures and nuggets buried in His Word."

Mike listened without saying anything. "I have heard others say heaven will be full of God's glorious creations, plants, animals, colors, and smells. I imagine flowers and trees will be waving and singing, too, with spectacular colors never seen before, changing colors with each new chord. People will be raising and waving their hands high, singing in complete harmony with nature, and worshipping the God who prepared all of this for us. And the music, Mike, we will be caught up with such richness, depth, and exhilaration. Our beings will participate in ways we never dreamed."

"Really?" He wanted to know more.

"We won't wear out praising the Lord! We will never be bored. It will never get old. But, on arriving to see Him, we will be unable to utter a single word because we will be so taken aback by all the glory, the complete peacefulness, and enveloping love. Tears of joy will flood our eyes, yet we will see clearly."

"It's hard to imagine."

"We will learn all the behind-the-scenes working of the hand of God in our lives and the times God plucked us from danger. We will be just like Abraham, who followed God's lead into a new land, even when Abraham did not comprehend all God had in store for him."

"Then why am I fighting so hard to stay alive if all of this is true about heaven?" Mike wondered.

I considered how to answer. I wanted Mike to stay strong and keep in the game. I reflected on how I trusted God, who is almighty, and in control of everything, even when events seemed to be going downhill in our lives. God knew this would happen and how it would happen.

"Let's just leave that at the feet of Jesus."

Being in Montana allowed us to reflect more objectively on our lives. We could see our lives more clearly looking from a distance.

"It will all be so perfect," I said. "And someday in heaven, we will meet the faith heroes of the Bible (Hebrews 11). We will get to talk with Abraham and Moses and David."

"Really?"

Mike loved hearing this because he had read about those Old Testament characters and their lives. When he read their Bible stories, we discussed how the Lord led them through trials and testing. God used and directed them for His purposes.

"Did you know Abraham is alive right now with Jesus?" I said.

"What?"

"Yes, there is a verse in the Bible that says, '*I am the God of Abraham, the God of Isaac, and the God of Jacob'? God is not the God of the dead, but of the living*'" (Matthew 22:31–32 NKJV). So the Abraham of the Old Testament, the one you admire so much for stepping out of his comfort zone to follow God to a new land, is alive right now with Jesus!"

"I never thought about that verse before in that way."

Quiet after that conversation, I mulled over how easily this conversation had occurred. Mike was quiet, too.

Could this be his last Montana visit?

MONTHS | *MAY 2017*

Back in Minnesota, as we tried to maintain as much normalcy as possible, I saw the changes in Mike; he sometimes needed help with balance. I had to take his arm to support him as we walked through airports, at the store, and in shops. Weaker now and tired all the time, Mike was due for another clinic visit. A year had passed since the doctor's awful "one year to live" statement and the conversation about where he wanted to die.

We had been to the clinic the day before to have Mike's blood drawn for the usual test. The test results, in my mind, were meaningless. *What did this test matter now that the ball was rolling down the hill with no return?*

We sat in the same tiny exam room when the doctor entered and greeted us with his usual warm smile and easy-going manner. Each visit was like seeing an old friend again. First, the doctor asked Mike how he was doing. How was he feeling? Was he still running? Then he gave us the news, "Mike, you have months to live."

I could see this crushed Mike. It shattered me, too. I knew Mike was going downhill, but I was not ready for this.

As usual, Mike negotiated with the oncologist, "Years?"

"Months. I wish I had better things to tell you, but you will have a pretty good summer."

As we went home, the news closed in on us. Neither of us spoke. Thoughts swirled in my mind. I felt unhinged from our regular life, suspended now to think things would not proceed as in the past. *It will be worse.*

We had heard the pronouncement before. However, a year had passed, and it had not come true. We both were stunned by these new words, perhaps me more than Mike. I had not allowed any thought of Mike leaving me. I had let the busyness of life float me, but now I was sinking under the news. I would actually have to swim, and I was not trained for that. I always had Mike to hang onto.

That night, Mike wrote in his running journal "THE NEWS."

Lord, this is hard. Be the sweetness in this bitter moment.

AUGUST 2017

Mike's doctor wanted to try one last chemotherapy. All too soon, however, we learned this therapy was a bust. Mike determined to go to Montana one final time. Up to this point, we spent time in Montana every few months between doctor appointments. Mike wanted to continue that schedule and still wanted to call the shots. As we visited the doctor and announced our plans, Mike described a new pain in his back.

"Let's do a scan and take a look. Then we will see about Montana."

After several days, we were back in the clinic to hear the doctor's verdict about our trip to Montana.

"The scan shows tumors in all but two thoracic vertebrae, and two tumors are impinging on your spinal cord." As he showed us the scans, he said, "Montana will have to be on hold for now."

Mike protested vigorously. "You mean you are forbidding me to go?"

"Yes, precisely that!"

"But I really want to go this one last time," Mike argued, knowing this would be his final trip there.

Exasperated with Mike's request, the oncologist told him the real truth. "This cancer could enter your spinal column, and all your limbs could become paralyzed! This could happen while you are in Montana. I cannot let you travel." Then he said, "Let's do radiation."

Despondent, Mike did not want to give up on his Montana trip. Quickly arranging radiation, the doctor ushered us out of the exam room. Our hopes carried us. The following day we drove downtown to the Radiation Oncology department, where we had been previously. All the same nurses welcomed us back. Radiation took fifteen minutes each day, and we were free to go until the next day's treatment. After one of these sessions, Mike exclaimed he wanted to go to the State Fair. How could I say no to his idea? Knowing his condition was questionable, and how unsteady he was on his feet, I went along with his request. I imagined we could get a riding cart for the Fair excursion. But upon arrival at the Fair gate, no riding carts were available. So, after three hours of walking and visiting Mike's favorite State Fair places, he was exhausted and ready to stop for the day.

I'M GOING TO RUN UNTIL I'M DONE

Several days after the end of the radiation series, Mike felt discomfort in his esophagus, so much so he did not want to eat or drink. I called the cancer clinic. They wanted to see him right away. They decided he was dehydrated and initiated a fluid infusion. We went home with ample liquid nourishment to tide him over the next few days.

The following morning, I inquired, "How are you?" expecting improvement. There was none. Mike had a fever, his esophagus still hurt, and he was coughing now. "Lord, help!" I pleaded. Not knowing what else to do, I drove him to the ER. Believing it to be an infection, the ER doctor prescribed antibiotics.

Mike's status did not change the next day. His temperature rose higher, his coughing continued. Upon calling his clinic and explaining the ER visit, and that Mike was now on antibiotics, they said, stay the course, "The antibiotics need time to work."

Wait! Wait! That is all everyone is saying! But things are not working! I could see the weekend approaching. At my wits' end to know how to proceed, I felt all alone trying to sort out what to do.

I called the radiation department and got the physician on call. He listened patiently to the sequence of events leading up to that time and decided Mike's deteriorating condition may be due to the radiation effect on his esophagus. "Continue with the antibiotics but call if he is not responding by Monday. *Everyone wants us to wait.*

At the beginning of the week, things were worse. I took Mike back to the ER. The doctor decided to admit Mike to the hospital to get his infection under control.

When I arrived in his hospital room, he looked so ill,

connected to all those bags of antibiotics and the oxygen tube. Over the next few days, his breathing worsened. The infectious disease team took cultures every six hours to discover the cause of his fever. Mike's oncologist stopped by to say he believed this episode was likely due to the cancer taking over Mike's body. *Oh! This is all moving too fast! This could be the end.* I emailed our church for our pastor to come.

I saw Mike was not improving. What could I do but pray over him? I read the verses I took with me everywhere—the fighting verses, the promise verses. It was my weaponry I brought to the hospital. "Lord, I need holding. I am helpless, except for You. I need to be carried right now. Lord, This is my crisis, too!" I read the verse, "*I am He, I am He who will sustain you. I have made you and I will carry you; I will sustain you and I will rescue you*" (Isaiah 46:4, NIV).

The following afternoon, our chapel pastor arrived at Mike's hospital room. I was sure he saw how Mike struggled for each breath, even with oxygen. He read the Scriptures and prayed over Mike. I thanked God for the comfort of this pastor and the comfort of the Word. Mike was struggling so hard to live.

Is this the end, God?

TURNAROUND | *SEPTEMBER 24, 2017*

As I walked into Mike's hospital room the following morning, Mike's breathing sounded more labored than the previous night. I scolded myself for not staying overnight with him. I had opted to sleep at home instead of on the window bench in Mike's room. *Mike could have died! What was I thinking?*

The infectious disease team arrived early and declared all

cultures were negative. Every few hours since Mike's arrival, they had taken cultures. They were now saying Mike's condition was not due to an infectious agent and told me the gamut of organisms they tested. I observed the questions on everyone's faces because they still had no diagnosis after three days. So, this team now turned the case over to the original doctors.

After the team left Mike's room, a clinical nurse arrived and reviewed their conclusion. We were back to square one. No diagnosis. "Could this be due to radiation?" I asked. "The radiation oncologist thought Mike's esophagus problem might be due to his radiation." She ran to the doctor's station just outside Mike's room. Within minutes, they ordered a potent anti-inflammatory drug to combat the possible radiation damage to Mike's lungs. Within two hours, Mike's eyes opened, and his breathing improved. I raised my hands to God who heals! One of my verses said it all! *"They cried to the Lord in their trouble, and he delivered them from their distress. He sent out his word and healed them, and delivered them from their destruction"* (Psalm 107:19–20, ESV). Another divine intervention in Mike's life! *To radiation pneumonitis, you mountain, you are thrown into the sea!*

Progressively Mike improved. By Tuesday, our senior pastor arrived. Shocked to see how well Mike was doing, this senior pastor relayed how the chapel pastor had told him Mike might not survive the weekend, but now he was alert, talking, and smiling. How sweet and upbeat was our visit! I shared the promise verses I brought to the hospital with our pastor and then silently praised God for Mike's recovery from this crisis.

Our pastor asked Mike if he had any questions. I could tell Mike was reflecting on his near-death status. "Is cremation biblical?" he asked.

"It does not matter. God does not need our old bodies to give us new bodies."

Then Mike asked his main question. "Do you remember what I asked you in Israel?" Mike reviewed with him about remarrying us at the Cana marriage site, where Jesus turned water into wine, and that the pastor had baptized us in the Jordan River. Mike wanted assurance that our pastor would fulfill his commitment to do his funeral.

"Of course, it will be my great honor."

That time seemed much nearer now.

---

1. Dr. David R. Reagan. "Applying the Science of Probability to the Scriptures," accessed 12/7/20, https://christinprophecy.org/articles/applying-the-science-of-probability-to-the-scriptures/
2. Chandra Wichramasinghe. "Evidence in the Trial at Arkansas, December 1981: What's New" accessed 12/7/20, www.panspermia.org/chandra.htm

4

THE FINISH LINE

CHANGES | *SEPTEMBER 27, 2017*

Every day the hospital floor hub outside my husband's room was Grand Central Station. Buzzing with doctors and nurses on computers or conferring with each other, I passed this station and headed for the family room at the end of this corridor. As I entered this empty room and closed the door, I found a quietness unknown outside that door. A massive stone fireplace commanded the space with floor-to-ceiling windows, capturing the downtown Minneapolis skyline. I watched as helicopters flew toward my windows, bringing sick ones to the roof above my husband's room. Today my peace would not be interrupted as it was the first time I saw helicopters flying directly at my window, then at the last moment, lift to land on the helipad above.

This fireplace corner room became my place to pray. With no one else in this room, I raised my hands. "Praise You, Lord, for bringing Mike through this crisis!" For the first time in five days, I allowed myself to relax a bit. After several moments of relishing in the peace of the moment, I returned to Mike's hospital room.

I took my usual seat on the wide window bench overlooking the grassy area below our eighth-floor window. Mike's oncologist popped into our hospital room. We had not seen him much through this crisis but heard his name paged over the speaker system several times. Both of us were delighted to see our old friend. He had come to discuss next steps.

"It is time to consider leaving the hospital," he started. He reviewed how Mike's lung problem was not due to infection or cancer but radiation. He said Mike would remain another day in the hospital, and then he would be released to continue on oxygen at home. Instead of being a celebratory session, this discussion turned in a direction we had not considered—hospice care.

Mike could not believe what he was hearing. "Surely, you have other things to try?" But the doctor explained he had no other treatment options. He had tried all the therapies in his armamentarium. Mike needed to be on oxygen, so his care had to accommodate this. I sensed Mike was anxious about being transferred to a different team and might no longer see his oncologist.

The doctor continued to present his case for hospice care. In the most comforting way, he described this care and the devoted people who delivered it as the best care available from a team specifically focused on Mike's needs—trained nurses, physicians, and others who would be available 24/7. This kind of care sounded like heaven to me. I spelled that relief! I would welcome relinquishing the pressure of trying to know what to do when Mike's status turned on a dime. Someone else would be calling the shots. The doctor explained that a nurse would visit twice weekly to manage Mike's symptoms and medicines and maximize his quality of life.

"Does anyone ever get out of hospice if they get better?" Mike queried because that was now his new goal.

"A possibility. Let's see how you do."

Hospice was the only option the doctor presented, so Mike reluctantly consented. I instantly felt the options narrowing, fencing us towards a gate of no return. We, however, were being carefully shepherded in this new direction.

Our oncologist offered, "Someone will be by to talk with you about this care." Mike grimaced, disappointed in this new direction.

Later that same morning, a hospice care manager arrived in Mike's room. Mike turned away from her in his bed. I motioned the lady to go to my corner fireplace room, my place of solace. There she explained the hospice program. Mike would no longer be under regular Medicare but under Medicare's hospice program, still paid for by the Medicare program. I saw the many papers she had for me to sign. *Whoa, Lord, is this new chapter the plan?*

She began by describing the care Mike would receive. "Mike will be getting a lot more attention and much better care in our program than if he went home under regular doctors' orders." She explained we would not be seeing Mike's oncologist anymore. Mike would not be seeing his primary care doctor either. We valued their care. However, more than this, we loved their friendship. These people were constants in our lives. Now severing those ties seemed heartless, a monumental loss. With each of Mike's doctors, we shared the excitement of seeing a mountain lion on our deck and a grizzly bear grazing in our back forest. They delighted in our stories. Now those ties were being cut—cruel at a time when we needed all the support and stability we could get.

Each doctor had their segment of care. Mike now required more focused and frequent attention. The new specialty team, comprised of doctors, nurses, and caregivers, focused its attention on Mike. The hospice manager described hospice care and concluded, "Hospice care is not only for patients who may be dying in days or weeks but for those who may recover some ability."

What a comfort. There might be a chance Mike could recover sufficiently and return to a prior status. I wanted days and months and, yes, years yet for him to live. As I signed the last papers, my solace room suddenly became chillier, and I now wanted to leave. I did not anticipate this hospice stage. I needed strength to carry on and be strong in the face of this transition for my Mikey. *Yes, the Bible said life is like a mist that quickly vanishes, but God, help us in this new season.*

HOME

More than ten years had passed since Mike's original diagnosis at age sixty-one. I was thankful for that time the Lord had given us. As this new phase began, I prayed, "Lord, help us. Help us accept Your will, Your way. This would not be our choice. Help us accept what is before us. And Lord, I need help, too, to get through this."

I left the family room where I had signed Mike into hospice and went back into Mike's room. I prepared to leave for home, gathering Mike's belongings and copies of the paperwork I had just signed. The coordinating hospice manager wanted me home before they delivered Mike and his oxygen gear. The oxygen van arrived soon after I came home, and the equipment was set up quickly by the front door. After about an hour, they delivered Mike attached to his portable tank. Our house quickly became a beehive with arrivals of supplies, drugs, and equipment. Within minutes, the rhythmic pumping of the oxygen compressor became the background noise for our home. The one-hundred-foot attached tubing became Mike's lifeline to allow ambulation to the farthest corners of our house.

The following day, a hospice nurse arrived for a get-to-know-you session. I immediately detected Mike's discomfort during this first session on our three-season porch. He wanted this visit to be quick and over. Her gentle manner soon won him over. But Mike warned her, still trying to make the rules, "I don't want an invasion of a lot of other people, only you." She had probably heard this before as she patiently listened to his directions. But, I already detected that her goal was Mike's best interests—his care, comfort, and quality of life. Gifted in the ministry of presence, she was there for him. *Thank You, Lord, for such caring, dedicated people!*

Mike's nurse, Laura, came twice a week; she was an absolute gem. Not only did she monitor Mike's medical condition, but she also sat and listened for as long as Mike wanted to discuss his situation or anything else. And talk he did, expressing how crushed he was at being in hospice. He voiced loss: loss of his regular doctors and their friendships, loss of treatment options, and loss of mobility outside the house and now tied to an oxygen line.

Anticipating Laura's return on the next visit, he was disappointed when a substitute arrived. They covered his needs—

medicines, oxygen, supplies, and equipment. As the nurse saw Mike required something new, she called in the order. Usually, deliveries came on the same day as the order. I loved that we had this care. I was relieved I did not have to make all the decisions anymore. I recalled his crisis days and how fretful I was about which doctor to call and what to do about Mike's quickly deteriorating condition. I thanked God for providing help.

Mike's damaged lungs began repairing from the radiation assault, and we anticipated continued recovery. Then, one day, a neighbor stopped by to visit Mike. Mike lamented he would like to be more mobile. She immediately offered to take him to the park in her fold-up wheelchair.

I could anticipate Mike's next request.

MOBILITY | *OCTOBER 2017*

His nurse fulfilled his wish with a new portable tank. He did not want to be constrained by the hundred-foot tube that tied him to the oxygen tank. With this new freedom, our neighbor wheeled him to Queensland Park for his first outing since the hospital, an event worth recording in his running journal.

Mike envisioned other outings like going for lunch at a café we liked in an adjoining town. These outings took time getting Mike and his gear in and out of the car. He was encouraged with each new step back to recovery, but I noticed his strength was waning.

Little did we know the "walk" to the park would be his last entry in his running log. It soon became evident he no longer had the strength to climb the stairs to our bedroom, a tremendous blow for him. I knew he was not about to be defeated by this. Envisioning solutions, he asked me to investigate installing a stair chair. Within days I found a company to install it. I helped him from the wheelchair into the stair chair so he could sleep in our bedroom. Solution! We both relaxed a bit with this new lift. The stair chair was a savior for me. Now I helped him maneuver from the wheelchair into the stair chair, reversing at the top. I no longer had to push Mike from behind, up every step.

One night as I began to lift Mike from his wheelchair onto the stair chair, he panicked. Screaming, he insisted, "You're going to drop me!" He demanded the help of someone stronger, our neighbor. Our wishes colliding, I reasoned we should not expect our neighbors to assist us with our daily chores. But Mike insisted. I reluctantly called our next-door neighbor, knowing this new complication would repeat itself several times daily. Our hospice nurse gave me a belt to help lift Mike at the next visit. Mike persisted I was not strong enough to move him. With no other alternative, I called the neighbors again.

HOLIDAY SEASON | *NOVEMBER 2017*

To the hospice nurse, I explained Mike's continuing insistence that I was not strong enough to move him. She took immediate charge of the situation and said to Mike, "It's time to get a hospital bed." Mike reluctantly consented. The first floor would be the extent of Mike's mobility.

The bed arrived the next day. Assembled, it took the space of half the family room. I was relieved we did not have to do the stair chair routine with Mike panicking. However, I also realized this was another step in a direction neither of us wanted.

Confined to the first floor, Mike asked me to buy a fish tank, something to view in his restricted living area. Mike recalled good memories of having a tank in his youth. I knew nothing about setting up an aquarium. Discovering what would be required took several hours. After skimming several websites and watching beginner YouTube videos, I ventured into inclement weather to purchase a tank and the accompanying paraphernalia. Within days I had the tank running and bubbling; after a few more days, we had eight fish. I positioned Mike near the fish tank in his wheelchair to enjoy the blue neons, guppies, a molly, and a swordtail. This lively dimension now graced Mike's confined territory. I loved Mike's drive to persevere. It helped me cope and covered the ache inside me that said this was temporary ground.

During this time, our next-door neighbor came to our home to talk and share stories with Mike. He brought yummy homemade soups every visit, each better than the last. The holiday season was approaching, and Mike wanted activities to happen for us, even though he was not ambulatory. As usual for this time of year, catalogs flooded our mailbox. These became a substitute for Mike's window on the world. Even in his debilitated state, he ordered Christmas decorations, candy, and gifts in an ordering frenzy, with packages arriving every few days. We usually erected our tall Christmas tree in the study with its nine-foot ceiling. This year, I bought a small fresh tree and placed it in the corner of the family room so Mike could view it from his bed. It warmed our spirits and assured some continuity in our fast-changing scene.

For years, my sisters and spouses exchanged names for Christmas gifts. My brother-in-law, Dan, had Mike's name for that year. He asked Mike what he wanted at one recent visit, knowing Mike may not have long to live. "A Wisconsin Badger hoody sweatshirt!" Mike blurted out. Back home in Wisconsin, Dan quickly ordered that gift and had it delivered Fed Ex. Upon receipt, Mike tried it on, then folded it up. He knew he would never get to wear it, but Dan would surely love it.

One day, a surprise! Mike's oncologist rang the doorbell, thrilling us with this out-of-the-blue happening! His presence lifted our souls, and Mike's face brightened to see his old friend. The oncologist leaned close to Mike and inquired about his symptoms and abilities. Mike talked about his loss of mobility, his "achy-breaky" pains, as he called them, and no longer being able to go to Montana one last time. Then, Mike showed the doctor his bandaged hand from thinned skin ripped open when he turned over in bed one night. Due to anti-clotting medications, blood continued to seep through each new bandage.

Patiently the doctor listened as Mike expressed, "I do not like where I am, but I accept it."

"Do you have any questions about how you are doing or about the dying process?"

Mike was taken aback at those last words, so the doctor unfolded, "You will sleep more and more, and in the end, you will die peacefully."

Mike listened, then blurted out, "When I go to heaven, I will meet Abraham, Moses, and David!"

"Yes," the doctor agreed with Mike.

Yes, and he will meet Jesus, too! I just don't want to think how soon.

INSTRUCTIONS

After this visit, Mike asked me to visit cemeteries and choose one. Online I searched for those that were close to our home. I wanted to get a feel for them, knowing someday this would be my final earthly place, too. I found one near our church and made phone inquiries. Meeting with the cemetery manager the next day, I wrote him a check for two plots. I was in a hurry.

At home, Mike asked me to meet with a funeral home to take pictures of caskets so he could choose his. At his direction, I planned and paid for the funeral costs. Mike specified he wanted two bouquets at his funeral, a red heart and a white cross. Precisely to Mike's wishes, I scrambled now to accomplish these tasks, during which time I pushed his death far out of my mind. He kept inquiring if I would be able to manage without him. Each time I assured him I would, not wanting him to know I had not allowed myself one single minute to consider this.

"Bring me some of those nice cards we bought in Montana," Mike requested. He wanted to thank his doctors, especially his oncologist and primary care physician. Writing in his usual block printing, he thanked them for their expert care during his life and for their friendship.

Mike knew a visit to his beloved Montana was off-limits, so he called friends in Montana and, in tears, told them how much he appreciated their time together and their help over the twenty years we had a place there. "I also want to give my nice knives to several people," Mike said. At our Montana home, Mike had a collection of knives. He recalled each one by maker and description. "Write down which one goes to each person." I could see he was tidying up even the small details as he was preparing to leave.

Our family room became a congregating place. I loved how our neighbors kept up their visits to chat, share stories, and bring the outside's happenings into a room Mike could not leave. One day, an entire family from across the street visited Mike and relayed something extraordinary. In finding their own home on Google Earth, their two young sons saw that the satellite's camera had forever captured Mike running on Eighth Avenue, around the corner from our home. *Just the way Mike would want to be remembered.*

DAYS | *DECEMBER 18*

Through all this time at home, Mike was preparing for leaving. I could see his complete peace with his situation. He believed the verse, *"You keep him in perfect peace whose mind is stayed on you, because he trusts in you. Trust in the Lord forever, for the Lord God is an everlasting rock"* (Isaiah 26:3–4, ESV). Because of this certainty, Mike had no concern about dying. His reservation in heaven was sealed. Nothing could change that. Only God knew the actual appointment time.

Several years earlier, he had written a note in his block printing that said, I KNOW HEAVEN IS FOR REAL. Mike had all things settled with God. Reiterating that we should live so we can throw off life like a loose outer garment at a moment's notice, Mike said we should be ready to leave this earth and live with Jesus after death. He understood he would have complete healing in heaven. God's purpose for him now was to hold onto the promises of the Scriptures of Jesus conquering death.

I became aware of Mike's conundrum as he became less conversive: should he stop fighting and give in, or should he wrestle to the end? This decision was not his. Mike started to sleep more of the time, and I began administering pain medication as drops into his mouth. I drew comfort in knowing, *"My [Mikey's] times are in your hand"* (Psalm 31:15, ESV). I changed my sleeping arrangements and brought an air mattress from a closet to sleep near him. I listened to his breathing to determine when he became restless. The doctor had told me restlessness might indicate Mike needed more pain medication. Like clockwork, I awoke every two hours to check on his breathing. Sleep-deprived and energy-depleted, I just went through the motions. Watching my husband dying was heart-wrenching, his once invincible spirit slowly fading.

During intervals in caring for Mike, I continued mindlessly knitting dozens of prosthetic breast inserts for cancer patients, a project for an organization called "Knitted Knockers." I learned about this project from a Montana friend several years earlier. I followed the habits of my mother and grandmother in keeping our hands busy even when we were sitting. Perhaps this was in denial of Mike's condition. He now slept around the clock.

On Tuesday, our favorite hospice nurse, Laura, arrived. I sat at the kitchen table, looking into our family room as she slipped the oxygen saturation clip on Mike's finger. She frowned as the device's alarm triggered. Her quick removal of it from his finger told me more than I wanted to know. She checked his feet and then came close to me with her assessment.

"Mike has days to live."

Like Mike bargaining with his oncologist, I said, "Weeks?"

"Days," she said.

I so wanted this not to be true.

CROSSING OVER | *DECEMBER 20*

Morning came on the twentieth. My waking every two hours left me sapped of energy. I recalled the words of the nurse the day before. After going through the motions of daily chores and caring for Mike, I sat down in a chair by his side, knitting, numb to everything else. Suddenly I heard Mike take a huge breath. *Is this his last breath? Why haven't I been paying attention to him? Why haven't I been by his side talking to him? Why haven't I been singing to him like my sister did when my mother died?* I railed at myself for being mentally absent when I should have been wholly present.

I rushed to his bedside and stroked his brow. I encouraged him, "It's okay. It's okay, Mikey," I cried. "It's okay to let go and be with Jesus." He took another huge breath. I was sobbing now, realizing the moment was here. "It's okay to let go and be with Jesus." And with a third breath, he did so.

Tears ran down my face. I continued stroking his brow. One minute he was breathing; now, there was silence and stillness. This discontinuity was complete and utterly alien. Engulfed in sobbing, I, too, was lifeless. Still frozen in my stance, leaning over his now lifeless body, I faced the moment I could not bring myself to envision before—life without my Mikey.

Overcome with tears but also fullness, a great peace settled over me. "My Mikey just met his Savior! In this auspicious moment, Mike just learned the meaning of his own name, Michael: *"Who is like Yahweh?"* I tried to imagine what joy now filled Mike's being. At that moment, Mike crossed over to be with Jesus in heaven. I had to release him and let him be there. I now had to take great joy; God's hidden hand had guided him safely there. He completed his purpose. This was his divine appointment.

I then thought about the fact Mike was not dead. *He skipped right over death into the arms of Jesus—a profound moment, a most sacred moment.*

A brand-new thing happened right before me. I had never been present when someone died. *Mike is set free of his earthly tent, minus his diseased body, ruined lungs, and cancerous spine. Cancer lost its battle to live; it had to die. But my Mikey is alive!*

At this moment, I knew my husband had just experienced there is no death! No death at all! *"O death, where is your sting"* (1 Cor. 15:55, ESV). To be absent from the body is to be present with the Lord. Jesus conquered death (John 11:25).

I was crying for joy and also for relief! My husband's struggle was over. Yet I could not move from him, wanting to savor this extraordinary moment: Mike's earthly life is complete. He is Home. He is now basking in the absolute fullness of joy and pleasures forevermore. I thought of the verse in Psalms; *"You make known to me the path of life; you will fill me with joy in your presence, with eternal pleasures at your right hand"* (Psalm 16:11, NIV). Mike fought the good fight, he finished his course, and he kept the faith (2 Timothy 4:7, KJV). Those Bible promises he counted on are happening. He's probably running a victory lap right now! The cancer is dead, but Mike is alive! So alive is he without his paralyzed left arm and chin, and he is living with perfect hearing and mobility. He is running and skipping and dancing in heaven.

I wish I could see the complete wholeness that captivates him right now and the overwhelming presence of Jesus with all that love and peace surrounding him.

The preciousness of the moment welled up in my soul. Tears flowed freely down my face. I did not even bother to wipe them as they dropped to the floor. At the same time, I began to recognize the deep, gaping wound inside of me.

INTERVAL

For an entire fifteen minutes, I could not break from Mike's bed to call hospice. Finally calling them with tears pouring down my face, I told them, "My husband just died." They offered their condolences and said someone would be over soon. Crying uncontrollably, I could not get out another word; I just hung up the phone. Overpowering emotions gushed from where I did not know. I was not an emotive person.

So full of joy and praise for Mike's home-going moments before, the intense loss now slammed me. Alone, I dropped onto the only remaining chair in the family room—Mike's chair—and sunk into hollowness.

Not moving for some time, I finally arose to switch off the ever-droning oxygen compressor. A stunning silence filled the house. Not prepared for this vacuum, there had always been noise in the house that represented life was going on here. But now, there was nothing. New and deafening. I was not sure I liked it.

Within ten minutes, I welcomed one of the hospice workers who usually bathed Mike. She was close by, and until our regular nurse could arrive, she offered me comfort and support. We talked and cried, sharing stories about Mike.

Soon our home became a hubbub of activity. Within the

half-hour, I emailed my close neighbors. They dashed over, not believing Mike had left so soon. I knew my sister and brother-in-law were also en route from Wisconsin, a visit they had previously planned to see Mike. They surmised by all the cars in the driveway that something had happened. They missed Mike's crossing over by a half-hour.

A time for crying and hugging, it felt as it should be—Mike's home-going, a precious event. *"Precious in the sight of the Lord is the death of his saints"* (Psalm 116:15, NIV).

Yes, he is safely home in the arms of Jesus!

I watched as the funeral home workers wheeled Mike out, and then other workers arrived to clear out the hospital bed, the oxygen equipment, and more. The house quickly emptied. Only the stair chair remained as a silent reminder of the life lived here. *My Mikey has gone ahead, and I am left here to deal with the pieces. God, I need You now, more than anything! Help me, Jesus!*

That afternoon I contacted the church office about planning the funeral. It was Wednesday and just a few days before Christmas. Hearing a voicemail, I left a message. The next day, the church funeral planner returned my call. She offered condolences but told me the church offices were closing that very day, and most people were leaving for the holidays. She described the implausibility of scheduling a funeral before the first week of January.

"At least we should find a date when the pastor is available and get the funeral scheduled. The earliest date is the third of January," she offered.

With the funeral date settled, my sister and husband stayed a day more and then returned to their home for Christmas family gatherings.

I have breathing room. I needed some space to gather myself together.

HOLE-IN-MY-HEART

Drained from Mike's round-the-clock care, I could not hold back the emotions flooding me. Life as I knew it shut down. Gone was everything I counted on: the companionship, the cheerleading, the sharing, the conversation, and the never-ending encouragement. All wiped out in the seconds of death. The hole in my heart screamed at me.

I sat in the very room where Mike died. I now faced complete emptiness. I never allowed myself to consider this stage. I had blocked thinking about Mike's death, keeping it out of bounds while caring for him, but the finale overtook me. Me, the planner!

Christmas Eve came four days after Mike's passing. I sat in the family room with a single lamp spreading its rays on the already dark evening. I felt enclosed in a cocoon. Suddenly it came to me. "I have to get out of this house! I have to get out of here." I was whispering. *Am I actually talking to myself? When did I start whispering?*

This is Christmas Eve. The stores are all closed. Everyone is with their families tonight. I am all alone. Why does this scene not compute?

I had the sudden urge to be in the company of others. Then, with computer-like speed, my mind quickly landed: *Go to the Christmas Eve service.*

I donned my winter coat and ventured into the snowy evening. In great exhaustion and emotional drain, I drove the fifteen miles to our church. Tied to Mike's 24/7 care in our family room for the last several months, I almost felt guilty for escaping.

Not a minute before the service began, I slipped into a balcony seat. The church was packed. I could be anonymous in the balcony and not have to speak with anyone. As I settled into my seat, the great organ swelled to fill the place with chords of "O Come, All Ye Faithful." We rose to sing. I felt I had been whispering for so long at home that I questioned if I still had a voice.

The music buoyed my sunken heart. But I could not sing. Nothing was there to help me get the words out. I just listened. Everyone was celebrating the joy of the season. Enveloping me like a warm covering, I allowed the songs and worship to minister to my hurting soul. Being in the presence of other believers and singing about our Savior coming to earth—this One who offered redemption to anyone who would believe and trust in Him—was salve to my soul this night. I knew my Mikey was present with Him at this Christmastime. The joy of the service did not seem out of place.

Upon their entrance to the sanctuary, everyone received a small candle with instructions that attendees would light these candles at the sermon's end. At that time, the auditorium lights turned low, and the place became aglow with a sea of tiny dancing white lights. At the same time, the organ swelled with the opening strains of Silent Night, then went silent as the leader led the congregation in singing a capella. I heard four-part harmony close around me, people enraptured in the experience as I was. I wanted to bottle this peace, this joy—this silent night, this holy night.

I raised my iPhone and captured the moment.

VIEW

I sat home for the next few days before the funeral, emotionally walloped, pondering life and how unprepared I was for Mike's leaving. As I began to process the previous days, I took to journaling. I thought about Mike in heaven. *He is alive right now.* Penning a song I hoped could be sung at his funeral, I envisioned Mike singing this song back to us from heaven.

> *Because of Jesus' death for me,*
> *I have new life eternally.*
> *My earthly life, O, it is done,*
> *And no more battles to be won.*
>
> *And now, with Jesus, I am safe.*
> *One day you'll meet Him face to face.*
> *O, friend, uphold the Word as truth,*
> *Throughout your life, you live on earth.*
>
> *I ask, O, death, where is your sting?*
> *I am alive, and I can sing,*
> *With throngs before me, I join in,*
> *At Jesus' feet and sing to Him.*

Still numb and exhausted at the visitation and funeral service on January third, I listened as neighbors talked about Mike's generosity and compassion throughout his life. I never knew what compassion looked like until I met Mike. How often did I see him stop and offer meals to homeless street people? Mike always said, "But for the grace of God, I could be in the same situation." Giving money to street corner beggars who would probably spend that money on booze or drugs, Mike would say, "God wants our hearts. Don't be concerned about how they spend it. It's what's in our heart that is important."

Mike's brother spoke about Mike's gift as a golfer. The pastor relayed the joke Mike told him while in the hospital. "There are no rain delays in heaven. Actually, there will be no golf at all in heaven because there will be no weeping and gnashing of teeth."

The solo song I chose for the funeral proclaimed that one day, we will all be rejoicing in heaven: *"When we all see Jesus, we'll sing and shout the victory!"* Yes, such a glorious day for Mike, and one day it will be a glorious shouting day for me, too. I had asked our pastor to read what R. C. Sproul wrote about death:

> When we close our eyes in death, we do not cease to be alive; rather, we experience a continuation of personal consciousness. No person is more conscious, more aware, and more alert than when he passes through the veil from this world into the next. Far from falling asleep, we are awakened to glory in all of its significance. For the believer, death does not have the last word. Death has surrendered to the conquering power of the One who was resurrected as the firstborn of many brethren.[1]

Shivering either from the chilliness of the chapel or else exhausted to the limit, I sat in the front row, listening to our pastor go through the promise verses I had given him when he visited Mike in the hospital. Mike and I had discussed those verses during his ten years with cancer. I was barely listening because I knew them inside and out. Instead, my mind wandered to Mike's struggle for these ten years. It was a miracle he even lived that long with such serious cancer. I thought those ten years were a time of testing our faith.

Perhaps all of life is a test.

FINAL CHAPTER | *JANUARY 2018*

The burial service day arrived. My sister and her husband returned from Wisconsin to be with me for this service. The day before, I had bought a single long-stemmed peach-colored rose for the service and stored it in my empty refrigerator. With no food in the house, I chose a restaurant nearby. As snow fell heavily, we pulled into the restaurant's vacant parking lot, which looked like someone had recently cleared it of five inches of snow. We ordered and dined, and as we were finishing, the waiter came to say they were closing for the night due to the snowstorm. As we left the restaurant, we realized five more inches of new snow had accumulated while we ate. I wondered about the burial service the next day.

The following morning, the funeral home called. "Can we postpone until tomorrow? Our hearse got stuck in another cemetery."

"Yes, of course." I had all the time in the world.

The following day came with the sun shining brightly and the cemetery covered with dazzling new snow. No need for the customary canopy over the grave. What a perfect day and a perfect way to remember the love of my life and my best friend. *Today is the day I bury my Mikey in the casket he chose. My husband of forty-two years is in more dazzling light at this moment than I can ever imagine.*

I thought of my Mikey, who, like Abraham, trusted God

wholly to carry him through his life. *Mike stepped out of his known world to follow God to a new land; there, he is alive right now!*

And I wondered if he had met Abraham yet.

---

1. R. C. Sproul, "Death Does Not Have the Last Word," Ligonier Ministries, Tabletalk Magazine, October 1, 2011.

AFTERWORD
NEW BEST FRIEND

Returning to my empty home after the service, I entered my study, where I met with God every morning. My seared heart searched for solace. I knew God said in His Word that He never leaves us; He is always with us—comfort words. I knew that truth all along. I knew the Holy Spirit took up residence in my redeemed spirit the moment I trusted Jesus as my Savior and Lord. The Holy Spirit was right there within me, waiting for me to recognize His Presence. He was Jehovah Shammah. *The God who is right here, right now.*

I gave Him my loneliness. *I want You to hold me, wrap Your arms around me, tell me I am whole, even though I feel halved.* As I gave this to Him, I realized I had Company, the Treasure within me without measure. I started talking to the Holy Spirit *(Ruach)* out loud. No more whispering.

And it came to me: *I now live alone, but I am not alone.*

I no longer asked why this ordeal happened to Mike, to us. I no longer questioned His ways, His timing. Though I could not understand everything, I trusted God was working all things out according to His economy—for His good pleasure.

As days passed, I had a myriad of decisions ahead of me, as outlined by my lawyer. With that long list, I gave them up to the Holy Spirit. *You take them; You lead me to handle everything.* To my inner Reservoir, I relinquished trying to run the show myself. I welcomed my Pilot-in-Residence.

I remembered what one of Mike's Montana friends said about Mike after his passing "I always liked being in Mike's space." *I wish I could be in Mike's space in heaven right now, just to glimpse the glory and experience the love that envelops him now.*

I thought about what it must be like to be in heaven, conversing with the Savior face to face. So one day, I asked the Lord, "Today, when You see my husband in heaven, would You call him Mikey?" I wanted my Mikey to know how greatly cherished and deeply loved he was. But I also knew he did not need more love than the Love surrounding him now.

About two months later, I asked my jeweler to find a green stone for my gold band—green to signify aliveness and life. He found the perfect tourmaline stone that now graces my gold band. I love to wear it to tell folks, "My Mikey is not dead, but alive with Jesus."

We asked Jesus for the miracle for Mike's healing, and He answered us. Those ten years living with metastatic cancer had not been about cancer at all.

DEAR READER,

Early in our understanding, my husband and I asked, "God, where are You in all of this?" and "Is this really Your best plan, Lord?" We struggled to find why He allowed cancer into our lives. Although we did not hear the answers to these exact questions, the Scriptures resounded with the message that God meets us in the hard places. He is there for us, saying, "You are not alone; I care deeply about you, and I will be with you through it all."

His big picture had us succeed according to His plan. As we camped on His Word, it spoke Truth and certainty into our souls. We felt covered with a blanket of His promises sewn together in a quilt made just for us. We abandoned our arguments and fears and let God's great peace settle over us.

I wish for you this story and these Words of Scripture lead you during your time of trial to find this kind of peace—His peace.

APPENDIX I
FIGHTING SCRIPTURES

The Word promises: With God, we can fight against any invader who destroys our peace.

"I will go in the strength of the Lord God."

— PSALM 71:16, KJV

"Stand firm and you will see the deliverance the Lord will bring you today.

— EXODUS 14:13, NIV

"Some trust in chariots and some in horses, but we trust in the name of the Lord our God."

— PSALM 20:7, NIV

"The Lord your God Himself fights for you."

— DEUTERONOMY 3:22, NKJV

"No weapon formed against you shall prosper."

— ISAIAH 54:17, NKJV

"Contend, O Lord, with those who contend with me; fight against those who fight against me!"

— PSALM 35:1, ESV

"They surrounded me on every side, but in the name of the Lord I cut them off."

— PSALM 118:11, NIV (1984 EDITION)

"The God of heaven will give us success."

— NEHEMIAH 2:20, NIV

"The battle is the Lord's."

— 1 SAMUEL 17:47, ESV

"With your help I can advance against a troop; with my God I can scale a wall."

— PSALM 18:29, NIV

"Surely the arm of the Lord is not too short to save."

— ISAIAH 59:1, NIV

"Those who trust in the Lord are like Mount Zion, which cannot be shaken but endures forever. As the mountains surround Jerusalem, so the Lord surrounds his people both now and forevermore."

— PSALM 125:1–2, NIV

"'I myself will be a wall of fire around it,' declares the Lord, 'and I will be its glory within.'"

— ZECHARIAH 2:5, NIV

"'Don't be afraid,' the prophet answered. 'Those who are with us are more than those who are with them.'"

— 2 KINGS 6:16, NIV

"There is no Rock like our God."

— 1 SAMUEL 2:2, NIV

"With You I can attack a barrier, and with my God I can leap over a wall."

— 2 SAMUEL 22:30, HCSB

"The weapons of our warfare are not carnal but mighty in God for pulling down strongholds, casting down arguments and every high thing that exalts itself against the knowledge of God, bringing every thought into captivity to the obedience of Christ."

— 2 CORINTHIANS 10:4–5, NKJV

"So do not fear, for I am with you; do not be dismayed, for I am your God. I will strengthen you and help you; I will uphold you with my righteous right hand."

— ISAIAH 41:10, NIV

"Trust that I AM; be not afraid."

— MATTHEW 14:27, JUB

"I will not die but live, and will proclaim what the Lord has done."

— PSALM 118:17, NIV

"Lord, save us! Lord, grant us success!"

— PSALM 118:25, NIV

"I have set the Lord always before me; because he is at my right hand, I shall not be shaken."

— PSALM 16:8, ESV

"God, who gives life to the dead and calls those things which do not exist as though they did."

— ROMANS 4:17, NKJV

"The Lord is my strength and song; he has become my salvation."

— PSALM 118:14, ESV

"At the name of Jesus every knee should bow, in heaven and on earth and under the earth, [*including prostate cancer*] and every tongue acknowledge that Jesus Christ is Lord, to the glory of God the Father."

— PHILIPPIANS 2:10–11, NIV

"The words that I have spoken to you are spirit and life."

— JOHN 6:63, ESV

"His divine power has granted to us all things that pertain to life and godliness."

— 2 PETER 1:3, ESV

"The Lord is faithful in all his words and kind in all his works."

— PSALM 145:13, ESV

Lord,

    Thank You that I can stand on Your Word, which is full of life and power. You are faithful to uphold Your Word and Your promises. You are with me now in my time of trouble. I am not afraid because there is no Rock like You. I will not be shaken. Your arm is not too short to save. The battle is Yours. I know You Yourself fight for me. Be a wall of protection around me. Contend with those who contend with me. Some trust in chariots and some in horses, but I trust in Your great name. As the mountains surround Jerusalem, so You, Lord, surround me now. I go forward in Your strength. No strategy is better.

    Amen

APPENDIX II
PROMISE SCRIPTURES

The Word promises: I need not fear. I need not be afraid.

"He who created you, O Jacob, he who formed you, O Israel: 'Fear not, for I have redeemed you; I have called you by name, you are mine. When you pass through the waters, I will be with you; and through the rivers, they shall not overwhelm you; when you walk through fire you shall not be burned, and the flame shall not consume you. For I am the Lord your God, the Holy One of Israel, your Savior."

— ISAIAH 43:1–3, ESV

"I, the Lord your God, hold your right hand; it is I who say to you, 'Fear not, I am the one who helps you.'"

— ISAIAH 41:13, ESV

"Fear not, for I am with you; be not dismayed, for I am your God. I will strengthen you, yes, I will help you, I will uphold you with My righteous right hand."

— ISAIAH 41:10, NKJV

"I sought the Lord, and he answered me and delivered me from all my fears."

— PSALM 34:4, ESV

"God is our refuge and strength, a very present help in trouble. Therefore we will not fear, even though the earth be removed, and though the mountains be carried into the midst of the sea."

— PSALM 46:1–2, NKJV

"He only is my rock and my salvation; He is my refuge; I will not be greatly shaken."

— PSALM 62:2, MEV

"Even though I walk through the valley of the shadow of death, I will fear no evil, for you are with me; your rod and your staff, they comfort me."

— PSALM 23:4, ESV

DEANA DICKERSON

"The Lord is my light and my salvation—whom shall I fear? The Lord is the stronghold of my life—of whom shall I be afraid?"

— PSALM 27:1, NIV

"Do not be afraid of them; the Lord your God himself will fight for you."

— DEUTERONOMY 3:22, NIV

Lord,
When I pass through the waters, You are with me; and through the rivers, they shall not overwhelm me; when I walk through the fire, I shall not be burned, and the flames shall not consume me, for You are the LORD our God, the Holy One of Israel, our Savior. I do not fear, for You are with me; I will not be dismayed, for You are my God; You will strengthen me, help me, and uphold me with Your righteous right hand. I do not fear because You are the one who helps me. I am not alone in this battle. You Yourself fight for me; I have only to believe. You are my refuge, my hiding place, my secret place. Lord, thank You for these promises.
Amen

The Word promises: Strength and protection for the battle when we trust Him.

"I have set the Lord always before me; because he is at my right hand, I shall not be shaken."

— PSALM 16:8, ESV

"The eyes of the Lord range throughout the earth to strengthen those whose hearts are fully committed to him."

— 2 CHRONICLES 16:9, NIV

"Those who trust in the Lord are like Mount Zion, which cannot be shaken but endures forever. As the mountains surround Jerusalem, so the Lord surrounds his people both now and forevermore."

— PSALM 125:1–2, NIV

"Trust in Him at all times, you people; pour out your heart before Him; God is a refuge for us."

— PSALM 62:8, NKJV

"Some trust in chariots and some in horses, but we trust in the name of the Lord our God."

— PSALM 20:7, NIV

"The Lord is good, a stronghold in the day of trouble; he knows those who take refuge in him."

— NAHUM 1:7, ESV

"Behold, God is my salvation; I will trust, and will not be afraid; for the Lord God is my strength and my song, and he has become my salvation."

— ISAIAH 12:2, ESV

"The righteous will never be shaken; they will be remembered forever. They will have no fear of bad news; their hearts are steadfast, trusting in the Lord."

— PSALM 112:6–7, NIV

"You are my refuge and my shield; I have put my hope in your word."

— PSALM 119:114, NIV

Lord,
You are the great I AM; You are ever-present even in my times of trouble. You never leave me or forsake me even when I am shaken. You are at my right hand. Just as the mountains surround Jerusalem, so You surround me now. You are good, a stronghold in the day of trouble. I have only You. I am in Your care, and I trust You will see me through this season. I am counting on You and Your great Name. There is power in Your Name, Jesus.
Amen

The Word promises: He will never forsake me. He will be with me through it all.

> "Be strong and courageous. Do not be afraid or terrified because of them, for the Lord your God goes with you; he will never leave you nor forsake you."
>
> — DEUTERONOMY 31:6, NIV

> "Have I not commanded you? Be strong and courageous. Do not be afraid; do not be discouraged, for the Lord your God will be with you wherever you go."
>
> — JOSHUA 1:9, NIV

> "I will bring the blind by a way they did not know; I will lead them in paths they have not known. I will make darkness light before them, and crooked places straight. These things I will do for them, and not forsake them."
>
> — ISAIAH 42:16, NKJV

> "I am with you always, even to the end of the age."
>
> — MATTHEW 28:20, NKJV

> "I am sure that neither death nor life, nor angels nor rulers, nor things present nor things to come, nor powers, nor height nor depth, nor anything else in all creation, will be able to separate us from the love of God in Christ Jesus our Lord."

— ROMANS 8:38–39, ESV

"I will never fail you. I will never abandon you."

— HEBREWS 13:5, NLT

Lord,

As an adopted child of God, I am promised You are with me continually. Even as I face this trouble, You are right here beside me. I need not be afraid. You are Immanuel, God with me. You are patiently waiting for me to recognize Your continual Presence. You never leave me or abandon me. I have only to speak aloud these verses to remind me I am never alone. Thank You, God, for these promises. Write them in my heart. Let me read them aloud! Let me recall them daily and, if needed, moment by moment. You are ever-watching; You are always available; You are unlimited, and You live in me. Let Your Word sustain me this day.

Amen

The Word promises: God does not lie. He keeps His promises.

"God is not a man, that he should lie."

— NUMBERS 23:19, ESV

"This truth gives them confidence that they have eternal life, which God—who does not lie—promised them before the world began."

— TITUS 1:2, NLT

"The Lord is trustworthy in all he promises and faithful in all he does."

— PSALM 145:13, NIV

"Not one word of all the good promises that the Lord had made to the house of Israel had failed; all came to pass."

— JOSHUA 21:45, ESV

"You know with all your heart and soul that not one of all the good promises the Lord your God gave you has failed. Every promise has been fulfilled; not one has failed."

— JOSHUA 23:14, NIV

"Praise be to the Lord, who has given rest to his people Israel just as he promised. Not one word has failed of all the good promises he gave through his servant Moses."

— 1 KINGS 8:56–57, NIV

"When God desired to show more convincingly to the heirs of the promise the unchangeable character of his purpose, he guaranteed it with an oath, so that by two unchangeable things, in which it is impossible for God to lie, we who have fled for refuge might have strong encouragement to hold fast to the hope set before us."

— HEBREWS 6:17–18, ESV

"I, the Lord, do not change."

— MALACHI 3:6, NIV

"He did not waver through unbelief regarding the promise of God, but was strengthened in his faith and gave glory to God, being fully persuaded that God had power to do what he had promised."

— ROMANS 4:20–21, NIV

"He who was seated on the throne said, 'Behold, I am making all things new.' Also he said, 'Write this down, for these words are trustworthy and true.'"

— REVELATION 21:5, ESV

Lord,

Thank You, You are faithful in all Your Words. Your Word says all the promises to the house of Israel came to pass. Not one word failed to come to pass. Thank You that You promised us eternal life. You are a God who never lies.

I can count on Your promises because You are able to do what You promise. You are THE promise-keeper. I can rest in all Your promises to me. What could be better?

Amen

The Word promises: His Word is total truth.

"The words of the Lord are pure words; as silver tried in a furnace on the earth, refined seven times."

— PSALM 12:6, NASB

"All Scripture is God-breathed and is useful for teaching, rebuking, correcting and training in righteousness, so that the servant of God may be thoroughly equipped for every good work."

— 2 TIMOTHY 3:16–17, NIV

"The sum of your word is truth, and every one of your righteous rules endures forever."

— PSALM 119:160, ESV

"You are God, and your words are true, and you have promised this good thing to your servant."

— 2 SAMUEL 7:28, ESV

"Lord, Your testimonies are completely reliable."

— PSALM 93:5, HCSB

"The law was given through Moses, but grace and truth came through Jesus Christ."

— JOHN 1:17, NKJV

"'I was born and for this purpose, I have come into the world—to bear witness to the truth. Everyone who is of the truth listens to my voice.'"

— JOHN 18:37, ESV

"Jesus said to the Jews who had believed him, 'If you abide in my word, you are truly my disciples, and you will know the truth, and the truth will set you free.'"

— JOHN 8:31–32, ESV

"Sanctify them in the truth; your word is truth."

— JOHN 17:17, ESV

"I am the way, and the truth, and the life. No one comes to the Father except through me."

— JOHN 14:6, ESV

"The Word became flesh and dwelt among us, and we have seen his glory, glory as of the only Son from the Father, full of grace and truth."

— JOHN 1:14, ESV

"All the promises of God find their yes in him. That is why it is through him that we utter our Amen to God for his glory."

— 2 CORINTHIANS 1:20, ESV

"Forever, O Lord, Your word is settled in heaven. Your faithfulness endures to all generations; You established the earth, and it abides. Unless Your law had been my delight, I would then have perished in my affliction. I will never forget Your precepts, for by them You have given me life."

— PSALM 119:89–90, 92–93, NKJV

"The grass withers, the flower fades, but the word of our God stands forever."

— ISAIAH 40:8, NKJV

"Scripture cannot be broken."

— JOHN 10:35, ESV

"This is the disciple who is testifying about these things and wrote these things, and we know that his testimony is true."

— JOHN 21:24, NASB

Lord,

I see it now: the sum of Your Word is truth. You represent absolute truth, total truth. The world has nothing better, nothing higher than that. The Word is God-breathed. That is so much better than man-breathed because God, You are the Almighty, the all-wise One. Your ways are higher than my ways. I can put complete trust in Your Word. Thank You for showing me that Truth came down to me. In Scripture, it says, in the beginning, was the Word, the Word was with God, and the Word was God. It also says the Word became flesh (Jesus) and dwelt among us. Jesus is God and the Word in bodily form, God with us. Jesus said, "I am the way, the truth, and the light. No man comes to the Father, but by me." There is no other way to have eternal life than accepting and trusting Jesus as Savior. The Truth is being made personal to me. Thank You for the power of Your Word and the Word of Your power.

Amen

The Word promises: Hope through healing.

"Praise the Lord, my soul, and forget not all his benefits—who forgives all your sins and heals all your diseases."

— PSALM 103:2–3, NIV

"Praise the Lord! How good to sing praises to our God! How delightful and how fitting! The Lord is rebuilding Jerusalem and bringing the exiles back to Israel. He heals the brokenhearted and bandages their wounds."

— PSALM 147:1–3, NLT

"He took on our infirmities and carried our sorrows; yet we considered Him stricken by God, struck down and afflicted. But he was pierced for our transgressions, He was crushed for our iniquities; the punishment that brought us peace was upon Him, and by His stripes we are healed."

— ISAIAH 53:4–5, NIV (1984 ED.)

"That evening they brought to him many who were oppressed by demons, and he cast out the spirits with a word and healed all who were sick. This was to fulfill what was spoken by the prophet Isaiah: 'He took our illnesses and bore our diseases.'"

— MATTHEW 8:16–17, ESV

"Have mercy on me, Lord, for I am faint; heal me, Lord, for my bones are in agony."

— PSALM 6:2, NIV

"They cried to the Lord in their trouble, and he delivered them from their distress. He sent out his word and healed them, and delivered them from their destruction."

— PSALM 107:19–20, ESV

"I will restore health to you, and your wounds I will heal, declares the Lord."

— JEREMIAH 30:17, ESV

"I will not die, but I will live and proclaim what the Lord has done."

— PSALM 118:17, HCSB

"The Lord is a refuge for the oppressed, a stronghold in times of trouble. Those who know your name trust in you, for you, Lord, have never forsaken those who seek you."

— PSALM 9:9–10, NIV

"I am the Lord, the God of all mankind. Is anything too hard for me?"

— JEREMIAH 32:27, NIV

"Listen to me...you whom I have upheld since your birth, and have carried since you were born. Even to your old age and gray hairs I am he, I am he who will sustain you. I have made you and I will carry you; I will sustain you and I will rescue you."

— ISAIAH 46:3–4, NIV

"My son, pay attention to what I say; turn your ear to my words. Do not let them out of your sight, keep them within your heart; for they are life to those who find them and health to one's whole body."

— PROVERBS 4:20–22, NIV

"'He bore our sins' in his body on the cross, so that we might die to sins and live for righteousness; 'by his wounds you have been healed.'"

— 1 PETER 2:24, NIV

"Do not be wise in your own eyes; fear the Lord and shun evil. This will bring health to your body and nourishment to your bones."

— PROVERBS 3:7–8, NIV

"Is any one of you sick? He should call the elders of the church to pray over him and anoint him with oil in the name of the Lord. And the prayer offered in faith will make the person well; the Lord will raise him up...Therefore confess your sins to each other and pray for each other so that you may be healed. The prayer of a righteous man is powerful and effective."

— JAMES 5:14–16, NIV

"This is how you should pray: 'Our Father in heaven, hallowed be your name, your kingdom come, your will be done, on earth as it is in heaven.'"

— MATTHEW 6:9–10, NIV

"Therefore I tell you, whatever you ask for in prayer, believe that you have received it, and it will be yours. And when you stand praying, if you hold anything against anyone, forgive them, so that your Father in heaven may forgive you your sins."

— MARK 11:24–26, NIV

"Until now you have not asked for anything in my name. Ask and you will receive, and your joy will be complete."

— JOHN 16:24, NIV

"He went throughout all Galilee, teaching in their synagogues and proclaiming the gospel of the kingdom and healing every disease and every affliction among the people."

— MATTHEW 4:23, ESV

"He came down with them and stood on a level place, with a great crowd of his disciples and a great multitude of people from all Judea and Jerusalem and the seacoast of Tyre and Sidon, who came to hear him and to be healed of their diseases. And those who were troubled with unclean spirits were cured. And all the crowd sought to touch him, for power came out from him and healed them all."

— LUKE 6:17–19, ESV

"Without faith it is impossible to please God, because anyone who comes to him must believe that he exists and that he rewards those who earnestly seek him."

— HEBREWS 11:6, NIV

"God, who at various times and in various ways spoke in time past to the fathers by the prophets, has in these last days spoken to us by His Son, whom He has appointed heir of all things, through whom also He made the worlds; who being the brightness of His glory and the express image of His person, and upholding all things by the word of His power, when He had by Himself purged our sins, sat down at the right hand of the Majesty on high."

— HEBREWS 1:1–3, NKJV

"Jesus Christ is the same yesterday and today and forever."

— HEBREWS 13:8, ESV

Lord,

You are my Creator and the Author of my life. You are the Healer and the Healing. For this, I am thankful and humbled. I bow before You. You said in Your Word that I must first ask forgiveness before I pray for healing. Right now, cleanse me of all sins, all wrongs I harbored, all wrong ways I went. Forgive my self-rule, my distance from You, and for thinking I can do life by myself. I give these up right now to You, the God Almighty, all-wise, who knows better than me what is best for my life. I thank You now for forgiveness.

I know You offer healing. In Your Word, You offer peace or shalom—meaning wholeness, completeness—spiritually, physically, and in our whole being. I know in the Garden of Eden, man began as being whole. But Adam sinned; after that, all humankind inherited a nature that was no longer whole. We became separated from You. We needed redemption, which You provided with Jesus— coming to earth as a man who gave His life in exchange for our sins so we could be made whole. Sickness, disease, and death entered the world at man's fall in the Garden of Eden. We must now deal with these consequences. You desire us to thrive, and we can use Your Word, which is alive and active, to thwart the enemy's plan. I continually pray the Word, bringing what You said in Your Word to You. You never change. You are the same yesterday, today, and forever. You healed in the past; You will heal today.

Your Word says the prayer of a righteous person is powerful and effective! I turn to You now and say back to You the promises of Your Word about healing. Your Word is Your power! Your Word is alive and active! As I speak these truths, I speak LIFE according to Your Word. You send forth your Word, and it heals me. Jesus took up my infirmities and carried my diseases. By Jesus' wounds, I am healed. You heal the brokenhearted and bind up my wounds. You save me from my distress. You rescue me from the grave. You declare You will restore me to health and heal my wounds. I will not die but live and will proclaim what You have done. I will not let Your words out of my sight; I will keep them within my heart, for they are my life and health.

You are the LORD, the God of all mankind. Is anything too hard for You? You will sustain me. You said, "Ask, and you will receive, and my joy will be complete." Be merciful to me, LORD, for I am faint; O LORD, heal me. I know You are a refuge for the oppressed, a stronghold in times of trouble. Those who know Your name will trust in You, for You, LORD, have never forsaken those who seek You. I ask in faith, nothing wavering, for without faith, it is impossible to please You. I come to You and believe You exist, and You reward those who earnestly seek You. I now bow to You, sovereign God. Your will be done on earth as it is in heaven. I pray all this in Your Name, Jesus.

Amen

The Word promises: His will is best.

"This is how you should pray: 'Our Father in heaven, hallowed be your name, your kingdom come, your will be done.'"

— MATTHEW 6:9–13, NIV

"My times are in your hand."

— PSALM 31:15, ESV

"I know that you can do all things, and that no purpose of yours can be thwarted."

— JOB 42:2, ESV

"He performs what is appointed for me, and many such things are with Him."

— JOB 23:14, NKJV

Lord,
I am completely and utterly hopeless on my own. I put You on the throne in my life.
My times are in Your hands. I bow to Your will. Let Your will be done in my life, I pray.
Amen

DEANA DICKERSON

The Word promises: Strength and help to endure.

"My flesh and my heart may fail, but God is the strength of my heart and my portion forever."

— PSALM 73:26, NIV

"Wait for the Lord; be strong, and let your heart take courage; wait for the Lord!"

— PSALM 27:14, ESV

"Our soul waits for the Lord; he is our help and our shield."

— PSALM 33:20, ESV

"May you be strengthened with all power, according to His glorious might, for all endurance and patience, with joy giving thanks to the Father, who has enabled you to share in the saints inheritance in the light."

— COLOSSIANS 1:11–12, HCSB

"Blessed is the man who remains steadfast under trial, for when he has stood the test he will receive the crown of life, which God has promised to those who love him."

— JAMES 1:12, ESV

"We count those blessed who endured. You have heard of the endurance of Job and have seen the outcome of the

Lord's dealings, that the Lord is full of compassion and is merciful."

— JAMES 5:11, NASB

Lord,

How can I live when the bottom has dropped out of my life? I am weak and have little energy to move forward. But God, You promised Your strength and Your power to sustain me and undergird me by Your power to continue living despite the circumstances. I thank You for upholding me and helping me endure with patience. Only by Your strength can I live. I depend on You for helping me through this season. You are with me to be my shield of protection, my strength for living, and my great Helper. Thank You for giving me the courage, patience, and endurance to get through this day. O, Lord, please don't leave my side.

Amen

DEANA DICKERSON

The Word promises: Comfort and care in our struggles.

"Cast your cares on the Lord and he will sustain you; he will never let the righteous be shaken."

— PSALM 55:22, NIV

"There is a friend who sticks closer than a brother."

— PROVERBS 18:24, ESV

"You, O Lord, are a shield about me, my glory, and the lifter of my head."

— PSALM 3:3, ESV

"I am he who comforts you... As a mother comforts her child, so will I comfort you."

— ISAIAH 51:12, 66:13, NIV

"The Lord is near to all who call on him, to all who call on him in truth."

— PSALM 145:18, NIV

"The Lord is close to the brokenhearted and saves those who are crushed in spirit."

— PSALM 34:18, NIV

"Casting all your care upon Him, for He cares for you."

— 1 PETER 5:7, NKJV

"But God, who comforts the downcast, comforted us."

— 2 CORINTHIANS 7:6, ESV

"Blessed be the God and Father of our Lord Jesus Christ, the Father of mercies and God of all comfort, who comforts us in all our affliction, so that we may be able to comfort those who are in any affliction, with the comfort with which we ourselves are comforted by God."

— 2 CORINTHIANS 1:3–4, ESV

"He will cover you with his feathers, and under his wings you will find refuge; his faithfulness will be your shield and rampart."

— PSALM 91:4, NIV

Lord,
 You say You are near to all who call on You. I call to You right now. You are the One who knows every detail of my life. You see every tear I cry. You know my heart and how much I hurt. You are the great I AM. I need Your closeness, Your Presence, Your comfort. Be the lifter of my soul; be the Friend that sticks closer than a brother. May these truths of Your Word sink deep in my heart and memory so that they come to mind every moment I need them. Help

DEANA DICKERSON

me get through this time when things are so bleak and I feel so exhausted. Cover me with Your wings. Wrap me in Your comfort. Hold me.

Amen

The Word promises: Peace.

> "You keep him in perfect peace whose mind is stayed on you, because he trusts in you. Trust in the Lord forever, for the Lord God is an everlasting rock."
>
> — ISAIAH 26:3–4, ESV

> "Peace I leave with you, My peace I give to you; not as the world gives do I give to you. Let not your heart be troubled, neither let it be afraid."
>
> — JOHN 14:27, NKJV

> "The peace of God, which transcends all understanding, will guard your hearts and your minds in Christ Jesus."
>
> — PHILIPPIANS 4:7, NIV

> "May God our Father give you grace and peace."
>
> — COLOSSIANS 1:2, NLT

> "God is not the author of confusion but of peace."
>
> — 1 CORINTHIANS 14:33, NKJV

> "Do not be anxious about anything, but in everything by prayer and supplication with thanksgiving let your requests be made known to God. And the peace of God, which

surpasses all understanding, will guard your hearts and your minds in Christ Jesus."

— PHILIPPIANS 4:6–7, ESV

"Unto us a child is born, unto us a son is given, and the government will be upon His shoulders. And He will be called Wonderful Counselor, Mighty God, Everlasting Father, Prince of Peace. Of the greatness of His government and peace there will be no end."

— ISAIAH 9:6, NIV

Lord,

Take away my fearful thoughts. I open myself to Your calmness, that peace beyond my comprehension. I focus on You right now, not on my problem. I hand over the controls to You. I take refuge right now under Your wings. Cover me with Your peace. Let it envelop me, rest on me.

Amen

The Word promises: Rest.

> "Come to Me, all you who labor and are heavy laden, and I will give your rest. Take My yoke upon you and learn from Me, for I am gentle and lowly in heart, and you will find rest for your souls. For My yoke is easy and My burden is light."
>
> — MATTHEW 11:28–30, NKJV

Lord,

I am overwhelmed. I need Your rest. I give You everything which is now in my life, all the changes, all the new demands, everything. I hand it over. You take it. I lay it at Your feet. Calm me, comfort me, settle me, soothe me, quiet me. Still my soul.

Amen

DEANA DICKERSON

The Word promises: I am of great value to God.

"The Lord your God is in your midst, a mighty one who will save; he will rejoice over you with gladness; he will quiet you by his love; he will exult over you with loud singing."

— ZEPHANIAH 3:17, ESV

"Then those who feared the Lord spoke with one another. The Lord paid attention and heard them, and a book of remembrance was written before him of those who feared the Lord and esteemed his name. 'They shall be mine,' says the Lord of hosts, 'in the day when I make up my treasured possession, and I will spare them as a man spares his son who serves him.'"

— MALACHI 3:16–17, ESV

"You are precious in my eyes, and honored, and I love you."

— ISAIAH 43:4, ESV

"God so loved the world that he gave his one and only Son, that whoever believes in him shall not perish but have eternal life."

— JOHN 3:16, NIV

"See what kind of love the Father has given to us, that we should be called children of God; and so we are."

I'M GOING TO RUN UNTIL I'M DONE

— 1 JOHN 3:1, ESV

"Precious in the sight of the Lord is the death of his saints."

— PSALM 116:15, NIV

Lord,

Thank you for creating me, giving me life, and placing great value on my life. I love that You treasure me. I love that You sing over me, and You love me dearly. You know everything, and You know I am going through a rough patch right now. You care deeply about me, as if I were the only person in this world. Let me hear You whisper these truths into my soul. Let me feel Your Presence, Lord.

Amen

DEANA DICKERSON

The Word promises: This earthly life is fleeting.

"Show me, Lord, my life's end and the number of my days; let me know how fleeting my life is."

— PSALM 39:4, NIV

"Man is like a breath; his days are like a passing shadow."

— PSALM 144:4, ESV

"My days are like a lengthening shadow, and I wither away like grass."

— PSALM 102:11, HCSB

"As for man, his days are like grass; he flourishes like a flower of the field; for the wind passes over it, and it is gone, and its place knows it no more. But the steadfast love of the Lord is from everlasting to everlasting on those who fear him, and his righteousness to children's children, to those who keep his covenant and remember to do his commandments."

— PSALM 103:15–18, ESV

"Moreover, no one knows when their hour will come."

— ECCLESIASTES 9:12, NIV

"You do not know what will happen tomorrow. For what is your life? It is even a vapor that appears for a little time and then vanishes away. Instead you ought to say, 'If the Lord wills, we shall live and do this or that.'"

— JAMES 4:14–15, NKJV

"All men are like grass, and all their glory is like the flowers of the field; the grass withers and the flowers fall, but the word of the Lord endures forever.' This is the word that was preached to you."

— 1 PETER 1:24–25, NIV

"Our days on the earth are like a shadow, and there is no abiding."

— 1 CHRONICLES 29:15, ESV

Lord,

Thank you for this life you gave me. The Bible says life is brief and is compared to a mist or a vapor. Help me understand life's brevity with a focus on the important things. Let me accept what is ahead. Let me envision the hope for the unimaginable glory I will experience in person with you someday.

Amen

DEANA DICKERSON

The Word promises: Physical death comes to all, but God provides a means to live forever with Him.

"In Adam all die, even so in Christ all shall be made alive."

— 1 CORINTHIANS 15:22, NKJV

"Just as people are destined to die once, and after that to face judgment, so Christ was sacrificed once to take away the sins of many; and he will appear a second time, not to bear sin, but to bring salvation to those who are waiting for him."

— HEBREWS 9:27, NIV

"And the dust returns to the earth as it was, and the spirit returns to God who gave it."

— ECCLESIASTES 12:7, ESV

Lord,

I am not looking forward to the dying process. I know as I pass through the veil of death, I will not die but go straight to be with you. You provided a way for me to be right with you, exchanging my sin with your righteousness, which guarantees I have eternal life forever with you. How can I thank you enough for this grand plan?
Amen

The Word promises: Jesus died, but He rose from the grave and is alive today.

"The angel said to the women, 'Do not be afraid, for I know that you are looking for Jesus, who was crucified. He is not here; he has risen, just as he said. Come and see the place where he lay."

— MATTHEW 28:5–6, NIV

"They were greatly perplexed concerning this, that behold, two men stood by them in shining garments. As they were afraid and bowed their faces to the earth, they said to them, 'Why do you seek the living among the dead? He is not here, but has risen! Remember how He spoke to you when He was still in Galilee, saying, 'The Son of Man must be delivered into the hands of sinful men, and be crucified, and the third day rise again.' And they remembered His words."

— LUKE 24:4–8, NKJV

"They rose up and returned to Jerusalem at once. And they found the eleven and those who were with them assembled together, saying, 'The Lord has risen indeed, and has appeared to Simon!' Then they reported what had happened on the way, and how He was recognized by them in the breaking of the bread."

— LUKE 24:33–35, MEV

"God raised him from the dead, and for many days he was seen by those who had traveled with him from Galilee to Jerusalem. They are now his witnesses to our people."

— ACTS 13:30–31, NIV

"He presented himself alive to them after his suffering by many proofs, appearing to them during forty days and speaking about the kingdom of God."

— ACTS 1:3, ESV

"I delivered to you first of all that which I also received: that Christ died for our sins according to the Scriptures, and that He was buried, and that He rose again the third day according to the Scriptures, and that He was seen by Cephas, then by the twelve. After that He was seen by over five hundred brethren at once, of whom the greater part remain to the present, but some have fallen asleep. After that He was seen by James, then by all the apostles. Then last of all He was seen by me also, as by one born out of due time."

— 1 CORINTHIANS 15:3–8, NKJV

"This Jesus, delivered up according to the definite plan and foreknowledge of God, you crucified and killed by the hands of lawless men. God raised him up, loosing the pangs of death, because it was not possible for him to be held by it."

— ACTS 2:23–24, ESV

"You will not leave my soul in Sheol, nor will You allow Your Holy One to see corruption. You will show me the path of life; in Your presence is fullness of joy; at Your right hand are pleasures forevermore."

— PSALM 16:10–11, NIV

"Do not be afraid, I am the First and the Last. I am the Living One; I was dead, and now look, I am alive forever and ever! And I hold the keys of death and Hades."

— REVELATION 1:17–18, NIV

Lord,

Thank You, Jesus, for not being a mere man, a good man, or just a prophet. God foreordained a plan to offer redemption to a fallen world through Your sacrifice on the cross. God sent You as His Son to become a man in an earth-suit, legally born into this world, yet sinless, to pay God's requirement for justice for my sin.

You completed God's plan to redeem sinful man. You did not stay dead but rose from the grave to live and reside at the right hand of God in heaven and in me. And not for me only, but for anyone who trusts and follows You. Who but You could have devised a plan like this? Thank You. I believe in You, my risen Lord.

Amen

DEANA DICKERSON

The Word promises: Death is conquered.

"He will swallow up death forever; and the Lord God will wipe away tears from all faces."

— ISAIAH 25:8, ESV

"I will ransom them from the power of the grave; I will redeem them from death. O Death, I will be your plagues! O Grave, I will be your destruction!"

— HOSEA 13:14, NKJV

"'Death is swallowed up in victory. O death, where is your victory? O death, where is your sting?' The sting of death is sin, and the power of sin is the law. But thanks be to God, who gives us the victory through our Lord Jesus Christ."

— 1 CORINTHIANS 15:54–57, ESV

"We know that Christ, being raised from the dead, will never die again; death no longer has dominion over him."

— ROMANS 6:9, ESV

"It has now been revealed through the appearing of our Savior, Christ Jesus, who has destroyed death and has brought life and immortality to light through the gospel. And of this gospel I was appointed a herald and an apostle and a teacher. That is why I am suffering as I am. Yet this is no cause for shame, because I know whom I have believed, and am convinced that he is able to guard what I have entrusted to him until that day."

— 2 TIMOTHY 1:10–12, NIV

"Since the children have flesh and blood, he too shared in their humanity so that by his death he might break the power of him who holds the power of death—that is, the devil—and free those who all their lives were held in slavery by their fear of death."

— HEBREWS 2:14–15, NIV

"We see Jesus, who was made a little lower than the angels, for the suffering of death crowned with glory and honor, that He, by the grace of God, might taste death for everyone."

— HEBREWS 2:9, NKJV

Lord,

death could not hold You! You surprised the enemy with Your plan of power over death. Death is fully and wholly conquered. You put death to death. It is the last enemy, and over it, You are victorious. You are the Almighty. Nothing is too hard for You. Death has no sting for me when I die. As a believer, I pass directly to be with You at my moment of death. Thank You for this great saving plan. Thank You for your Word that speaks life to me through the work on the cross. Help me remember the high price You paid in dying for me so I might have life now and eternally.

Amen

DEANA DICKERSON

The Word promises: Jesus is the firstborn from the dead.

"That the Christ would suffer, that He would be the first to rise from the dead, and would proclaim light to the Jewish people and to the Gentiles."

— ACTS 26:23, NKJV

"Christ has indeed been raised from the dead, the first-fruits of those who have fallen asleep. For since death came through a man, the resurrection of the dead comes also through a man. For as in Adam all die, so in Christ all will be made alive. But each in turn: Christ, the first-fruits; then, when he comes, those who belong to him."

— 1 CORINTHIANS 15:20–23, NIV

"Those whom he foreknew he also predestined to be conformed to the image of his Son, in order that he might be the firstborn among many brothers."

— ROMANS 8:29, ESV

"He is the head of the body, the church, who is the beginning, the firstborn from the dead, that in all things He may have the preeminence."

— COLOSSIANS 1:18, NKJV

"Grace and peace to you from him who is, and who was, and who is to come, and from the seven spirits before his throne, and from Jesus Christ, who is the faithful witness, the firstborn from the dead, and the ruler of the kings of the earth."

— REVELATION 1:4–5, NIV

Lord,

I love the promises in Your Word. It says Jesus died for my sins, but on the third day, He rose to live again, conquering sin and death. Your Word says He is the first to rise from the grave. You give me a future and a hope that believers will also rise. I can have great peace and rest in Your promise that I pass over death and rise to be with You. What comfort we have in You.

Amen

DEANA DICKERSON

The Word promises: I, too, will rise.

"Your dead will live, Lord; their bodies will rise—let those who dwell in the dust wake up and shout for joy—your dew is like the dew of the morning; the earth will give birth to her dead."

— ISAIAH 26:19, NIV

"Many of those who sleep in the dust of the earth shall awake, some to everlasting life, and some to shame and everlasting contempt."

— DANIEL 12:2, ESV

"Behold! I tell you a mystery. We shall not all sleep, but we shall all be changed, in a moment, in the twinkling of an eye, at the last trumpet. For the trumpet will sound, and the dead will be raised imperishable, and we shall be changed."

— 1 CORINTHIANS 15:51–52, ESV

"If we have been united with him in a death like his, we will certainly also be united with him in a resurrection like his."

— ROMANS 6:5, NIV

"You shall know that I am the Lord, when I open your graves, and raise you from your graves, O my people. And I will put my Spirit within you, and you shall live, and I will place you in your own land. Then you shall know that I am the Lord; I have spoken, and I will do it, declares the Lord."

— EZEKIEL 37:13–14, ESV

Lord,

This is extraordinary. I live after physical death! This life is not all there is, as many people think. I rise after passing through the veil of death to be with You, Jesus. You say You never leave me or forsake me. At no time are You not with me. Physical bodies may be in the grave until the end of the age until we all get new bodies, but our souls and spirits are alive with You. I am utterly speechless before You for the encompassing plan. I am so grateful and humbled to take part in Your plan.

Amen

DEANA DICKERSON

The Word promises: My mortal body may be wasting away, but my spirit is being renewed.

"We do not lose heart. Though our outer self is wasting away, our inner self is being renewed day by day."

— 2 CORINTHIANS 4:16, ESV

"We know that if the tent that is our earthly home is destroyed, we have a building from God, a house not made with hands, eternal in the heavens. For in this tent we groan, longing to put on our heavenly dwelling, if indeed by putting it on we may not be found naked. For while we are still in this tent, we groan, being burdened—not that we would be unclothed, but that we would be further clothed, so that what is mortal may be swallowed up by life. He who has prepared us for this very thing is God, who has given us the Spirit as a guarantee."

— 2 CORINTHIANS 5:1–5, ESV

Lord,

Help me remember that as my physical frame declines and aches and pains take over much of my thinking, my spirit is renewed daily, even though my body may be groaning with illness or disease. I have the guarantee by Your Word that someday I, too, will be loosed from this mortal body and have new life in eternity. Yes, I continue to pray for healing and help with my physical problems, but You are in charge. The more I hurt, the more I need You close to me. So help me focus on You, not my pain.

Amen

DEANA DICKERSON

The Word promises: I will have a new body.

"Our citizenship is in heaven, from which we also eagerly wait for the Savior, the Lord Jesus Christ, who will transform our lowly body that it may be conformed to His glorious body, according to the working by which He is able even to subdue all things to Himself."

— PHILIPPIANS 3:20–21, NKJV

"This perishable body must put on the imperishable, and this mortal body must put on immortality. When the perishable puts on the imperishable, and the mortal puts on immortality, then shall come to pass the saying that is written: 'Death is swallowed up in victory. O death, where is your victory? O death where is your sting?'"

— 1 CORINTHIANS 15:53–55, ESV

"Not only creation, but we ourselves, who have the firstfruits of the Spirit, groan inwardly as we wait eagerly for adoption as sons, the redemption of our bodies. For in this hope we were saved. Now hope that is seen is not hope. For who hopes for what he sees? But if we hope for what we do not see, we wait for it with patience."

— ROMANS 8:23–25, ESV

"This I say, brethren, that flesh and blood cannot inherit the kingdom of God; nor does corruption inherit incorruption.

> Behold, I tell you a mystery: We shall not all sleep, but we shall all be changed."
>
> — 1 CORINTHIANS 15:50–51, NKJV

I praise You, Lord,

Thank You for what Your Word tells me about the redemption of my body. My old diseased body will be forever gone. My new body will never die or decline, but it will be like Your glorious body, all accomplished with Your power. But I know this will not be my highest joy. Seeing You and basking in Your love will be my soul's delight.

Amen

DEANA DICKERSON

The Word promises: I will have life after this life.

"The Lord loves justice, and does not forsake His saints; they are preserved forever, but the descendants of the wicked shall be cut off. The righteous shall inherit the land, and dwell in it forever."

— PSALM 37:28–29, NKJV

"God will redeem my soul from the power of the grave, for He shall receive me."

— PSALM 49:15, NKJV

"Our God is a God who saves; from the Sovereign Lord comes escape from death."

— PSALM 68:20, NIV

"Therefore my heart is glad, and my tongue rejoices; my body also will rest secure, because you will not abandon me to the realm of the dead, or let your faithful one see decay. You make known to me the path of life; you fill me with joy in your presence, with eternal pleasures at your right hand."

— PSALM 16:9–11, NIV

"Bless the Lord, my soul, and forget not all his benefits…who redeems your life from the pit and crowns you with love and mercy."

— PSALM 103:2, 4, ESV

"In the path of righteousness is life, and in its pathway there is no death."

— PROVERBS 12:28, ESV

"Jesus said to her, 'I am the resurrection and the life. Whoever believes in me, though he die, yet shall he live, and everyone who lives and believes in me shall never die. Do you believe this?'"

— JOHN 11:25–26, ESV

"Truly, truly, I say to you, if anyone keeps my word, he will never see death."

— JOHN 8:51, ESV

"As in Adam all die, so also in Christ shall all be made alive."

— 1 CORINTHIANS 15:22, ESV

"Because I live, you will also live."

— JOHN 14:19B, NIV

DEANA DICKERSON

"Truly, truly, I say to you, whoever hears my word and believes him who sent me has eternal life. He does not come into judgment, but has passed from death to life."

— JOHN 5:24, ESV

"Concerning the resurrection of the dead, have you not read what was spoken to you by God, saying, 'I am the God of Abraham, the God of Isaac, and the God of Jacob'? God is not God of the dead, but of the living."

— MATTHEW 22:31–32, NKJV

Lord,

You are the resurrection and the life. Whoever believes in You, though he dies, yet shall he live. I will live with You after death! Right now, Abraham, Isaac, and Jacob are alive! The verse says, 'I am the God of Abraham, Isaac, and Jacob!' All believers who have died are also alive with You right now. Why would anyone not want this? I am delivered from death. I live beyond the existence of this earthly life. I have pleasures forevermore. Forever means F O R E V E R! My praise to You is so feeble compared to all You give me! How can I express my thanks in a way that honors Your enormous graciousness and mercy? I humbly lift my hands to You and bow my head before You. I know You inhabit my praise, so it is the least I can do in worshipping You.

Amen

The Word promises: When I physically die, I will be with Jesus.

"One of the criminals who were hanged railed at him, saying, 'Are you not the Christ? Save yourself and us!' But the other rebuked him, saying, "Do you not fear God, since you are under the same sentence of condemnation? And we indeed justly, for we are receiving the due reward of our deeds; but this man has done nothing wrong.' And he said, 'Jesus, remember me when you come into your kingdom.' And he said to him, 'Truly, I say to you, today you will be with me in paradise.'"

— LUKE 23:39–43, ESV

"We are always confident and know that as long as we are at home in the body we are away from the Lord. For we live by faith, not by sight. We are confident, I say, and would prefer to be away from the body and at home with the Lord. So we make it our goal to please him, whether we are at home in the body or away from it."

— 2 CORINTHIANS 5:6–9, NIV

"Brothers and sisters, we do not want you to be uninformed about those who sleep in death, so that you do not grieve like the rest of mankind, who have no hope. For we believe that Jesus died and rose again, and so we believe that God will bring with Jesus those who have fallen asleep in him."

— 1 THESSALONIANS 4:13–14, NIV

"Do not let not your heart be troubled; believe in God, believe also in Me. In My Father's house are many rooms; if that were not so, I would have told you, because I am going there to prepare a place for you. And if I go and prepare a place for you, I am coming again and will take you to Myself, so that where I am, there you also will be."

— JOHN 14:1–3, NASB

"God has not destined us for wrath, but to obtain salvation through our Lord Jesus Christ, who died for us so that whether we are awake or asleep we might live with Him."

— 1 THESSALONIANS 5:9–10, ESV

"When Christ who is our life appears, then you also will appear with Him in glory."

— COLOSSIANS 3:4, NKJV

"This saying is trustworthy: For if we have died with Him, we will also live with Him; if we endure, we will also reign with Him."

— 2 TIMOTHY 2:11–12, HCSB

"Knowing that he who raised the Lord Jesus will raise us also with Jesus and bring us with you into his presence."

— 2 CORINTHIANS 4:14, ESV

"I am hard pressed between the two. My desire is to depart and be with Christ, for that is far better. But to remain in the flesh is more necessary on your account."

— PHILIPPIANS 1:23–24, ESV

Jesus,

I thank You that I will be with You when I pass away from this earthly life. Your Word explains to be away from the body is to be at home with the Lord. Therefore, I will be immediately with You after my last millisecond of life on earth. My family does not need to grieve as others but should rejoice with Your Word's assurance that I am safely home with You. I love that thought.

Amen

DEANA DICKERSON

The Word promises: God can rescue me but even if He does not, I choose to serve Him.

"Shadrach, Meshach, and Abednego answered and said to the king, 'O Nebuchadnezzar, we have no need to answer you in this matter. If this be so, our God whom we serve is able to deliver us from the burning fiery furnace, and he will deliver us out of your hand, O king. But if not, be it known to you, O king, that we will not serve your gods or worship the golden image that you have set up.'"

— DANIEL 3:16–18, ESV

"Though He slay me, I will hope in Him…"

— JOB 13:15, NKJV

Lord,

Help me stand like Shadrach, Meshach, and Abednego in times of great trials. They knew if You chose not to rescue them, they were in Your hands and care. Even if they died in their great trial, they would still be with You in both life and death. They left it up to You and Your plan. They chose to have complete faith in You. Help me to remember You are with me always, even in my darkest trial. You are Jehovah Shammah, the God who is right here, right now. You can be trusted, no matter what happens. You never leave me or forsake me. Help me to stand strong. Strengthen my faith in You and the promises in Your Word.

Amen

The Word promises: In this world I will have trouble. But my affliction is temporary and is light compared to the glory to come.

"I have told you these things, so that in Me you may have peace. In this world you will have trouble. But take heart! I have overcome the world."

— JOHN 16:33, NIV

"In this you greatly rejoice, even though now, if for a little while...you have had to suffer various trials, in order that the genuineness of your faith, which is more precious than gold that perishes, though it is tried by fire, may be found to result in praise, glory, and honor at the revelation of Jesus Christ."

— 1 PETER 1:6–7, MEV

"Our light affliction, which is but for a moment, is working for us a far more exceeding and eternal weight of glory."

— 2 CORINTHIANS 4:17, NKJV

"I consider that the sufferings of this present time are not worth comparing with the glory that will be revealed to us."

— ROMANS 8:18, ESV

"Weeping may tarry for the night, but joy comes in the morning."

DEANA DICKERSON

— PSALM 30:5B, ESV

Lord,

Help me understand that my present afflictions are temporary. And help me see these trials are not worth comparing to the glory to come. Help me see that, at some point, I will be freed from this earthly tent and be in glory with You. I will have a new glorious body like Yours. I will see You face to face. But be with me now in my suffering. Give me Your piece to endure.

Amen

The Word promises: If I live or die, I am the Lord's.

"If we live, we live to the Lord, and if we die, we die to the Lord. So then, whether we live or whether we die, we are the Lord's. For to this end Christ died and lived again, that he might be Lord both of the dead and of the living."

— ROMANS 14:8–9, ESV

Lord,

Help me realize there is more to life than this life. Help me to understand there is life forever with You. I want to be more like Paul saying: I am with You in life or death. I believe Your Word.

Amen

DEANA DICKERSON

The Word promises: that heaven awaits me after death if I am a believer.

> "Our citizenship is in heaven, and from it we await a Savior, the Lord Jesus Christ, who will transform our lowly body to be like his glorious body, by the power that enables him even to subject all things to himself."
>
> — PHILIPPIANS 3:20–21, ESV

> "Let not your hearts be troubled. Believe in God; believe also in me. In my Father's house are many rooms. If it were not so, would I have told you that I go to prepare a place for you? And if I go and prepare a place for you, I will come again and will take you to myself, that where I am you may be also."
>
> — JOHN 14:1–3, ESV

> "The Lord will rescue me from every evil deed and bring me safely into his heavenly kingdom. To him be the glory forever and ever. Amen."
>
> — 2 TIMOTHY 4:18, ESV

> "Blessed are the poor in spirit, for theirs is the kingdom of heaven."
>
> — MATTHEW 5:3, NIV

> "You guide me with your counsel, leading me to a glorious destiny."

I'M GOING TO RUN UNTIL I'M DONE

— PSALM 73:24, NLT

"Blessed be the God and Father of our Lord Jesus Christ! According to his great mercy, he has caused us to be born again to a living hope through the resurrection of Jesus Christ from the dead, to an inheritance that is imperishable, undefiled, and unfading, kept in heaven for you, who by God's power are being guarded through faith for a salvation ready to be revealed in the last time."

— 1 PETER 1:3–5, ESV

"Nevertheless, do not rejoice in this, that the spirits are subject to you, but rejoice that your names are written in heaven."

— LUKE 10:20, ESV

"God, being rich in mercy, because of the great love with which he loved us, even when we were dead in our trespasses, made us alive together with Christ—by grace you have been saved—and raised us up with him and seated us with him in the heavenly places in Christ Jesus, so that in the coming ages he might show the immeasurable riches of his grace in kindness toward us in Christ Jesus."

— EPHESIANS 2:4–7, ESV

"We have heard of your faith in Christ Jesus...the faith and love that spring from the hope stored up for you in heaven and about which you have already heard in the true message of the gospel.

— COLOSSIANS 1:4–5, NIV

"'He will wipe every tear from their eyes. There will be no more death' or mourning or crying or pain, for the old order of things has passed away."

— REVELATION 21:4, NIV

"'Never again will they hunger; never again will they thirst. The sun will not beat down on them,' nor any scorching heat. For the Lamb at the center of the throne will be their shepherd; 'he will lead them to springs of living water.' 'And God will wipe away every tear from their eyes.'"

— REVELATION 7:16–17, NIV

"I create new heavens and a new earth, and the former things shall not be remembered or come into mind."

— ISAIAH 65:17, ESV

"Night will be no more. They will need no light of lamp or sun, for the Lord God will be their light, and they will reign forever and ever."

— REVELATION 22:5, ESV

> "You have come to Mount Zion and to the city of the living God, the heavenly Jerusalem, and to innumerable angels in festal gathering, and to the assembly of the firstborn who are enrolled in heaven, and to God, the judge of all, and to the spirits of the righteous made perfect, and to Jesus, the mediator of a new covenant, and to the sprinkled blood that speaks a better word than the blood of Abel."
>
> — HEBREWS 12:22–24, ESV

> "After this I looked, and behold, a door standing open in heaven! And the first voice, which I had heard speaking to me like a trumpet, said, 'Come up here, and I will show you what must take place after this.' At once I was in the Spirit, and behold, a throne stood in heaven, with one seated on the throne. And he who sat there had the appearance of jasper and carnelian, and around the throne was a rainbow that had the appearance of an emerald. Around the throne were twenty-four thrones, and seated on the thrones were twenty-four elders, clothed in white garments, with golden crowns on their heads. From the throne came flashes of lightning, and rumblings and peals of thunder, and before the throne were burning seven torches of fire, which are the seven spirits of God, and before the throne there was as it were a sea of glass."
>
> — REVELATION 4:1–6, ESV

Lord,

I love Your words about heaven. It will be so unlike earth it is hard for me to imagine. And best of all, I will be in Your presence, seeing Your face and worshiping You. You have a spot reserved for me in heaven. It is not mere wishful thinking but a virtual certainty. The Holy Spirit guarantees it. You promise this in Your Word, and Your Word is Truth. I have eternal life with You. How can I thank You enough for making it possible for puny me, who has made so many mistakes in my life, to have the assurance of heaven? I thank You for forgiving me of all my sins, canceling them out, and providing a way I can live with You forever. Glory!

Amen

The Word Promises: God is above all. Therefore I should praise Him for all His promises.

"Be still, and know that I am God."

— PSALM 46:10, NKJV

"The Lord is in his holy temple; let all the earth be silent before him."

— HABAKKUK 2:20, NIV

"How great you are, Sovereign Lord! There is no one like you, and there is no God but you, as we have heard with our own ears."

— 2 SAMUEL 7:22, NIV

"Sing to the Lord, for He has done excellent things; this is known in all the earth. Cry out and shout, O inhabitant of Zion, for great is the Holy One of Israel in your midst!"

— ISAIAH 12:5–6, NKJV

"Give to the Lord the glory due His name; bring an offering, and come before Him. Oh, worship the Lord in the beauty of holiness!"

— 1 CHRONICLES 16:29, NKJV

"Your steadfast love is better than life, my lips will praise you. So I will bless you as long as I live; in your name I will lift up my hands."

— PSALM 63:3–4, ESV

"Come, let us worship and bow down; let us kneel before the Lord, our Maker! For he is our God, and we are the people of his pasture, and the sheep of his hand."

— PSALM 95:6–7, ESV

"Praise the Lord, my soul; all my inmost being, praise his holy name. Praise the Lord, my soul, and forget not all his benefits—who forgives all your sins and heals all your diseases, who redeems your life from the pit and crowns you with love and compassion, who satisfies your desires with good things so that your youth is renewed like the eagle's."

— PSALM 103:1–5, NIV

"Exalt the Lord our God, and worship at His holy hill; for the Lord our God is holy."

— PSALM 99:9, NKJV

"Great is the Lord, and greatly to be praised, and his greatness is unsearchable."

— PSALM 145:3, ESV

"Jesus answered him, 'It is written, You shall worship the Lord your God, and him only shall you serve.'"

— LUKE 4:8, ESV

"To him who sits on the throne and to the Lamb be blessing and honor and glory and might forever and ever!"

— REVELATION 5:13, ESV

Lord,

I worship You. I surrender everything to You. You are holy. Honor, glory, majesty, dominion, and power are Yours. I lift my hands to You. I bow down before You. I am in awe of Your weightiness.

Amen

DEANA DICKERSON

The Word promises: I will give an account of how I lived my life.

"What will I do when God confronts me? What will I answer when called to account?"

— JOB 31:14, NIV

"Each of us will give an account of himself to God."

— ROMANS 14:12, ESV

"God will bring every deed into judgment, with every secret thing, whether good or evil."

— ECCLESIASTES 12:14 ESV

Lord,

I know everyone will have to give an account of their lives when we stand before You in heaven when the books are opened. For us who believed and received You as Savior, our sins have been erased, wiped clean, forgotten, and removed as far as the east is from the west. We have received mercy and grace. At that time, You reward our good deeds done for You. Those who do not believe and trust in You will receive justice. Thank You, I am counted righteous in Your sight. Oh, the price You willingly paid to redeem me. I have great peace and certainty about my future with You.

Amen

The Word promises: By repenting of my sins and believing in Jesus, who paid for my sins, I can be forgiven and have new life now and eternally.

> "God so loved the world, that he gave his only Son, that whoever believes in him should not perish but have eternal life. For God did not send his Son into the world to condemn the world, but in order that the world might be saved through him. Whoever believes in him is not condemned, but whoever does not believe is condemned already, because he has not believed in the name of the only Son of God."
>
> — JOHN 3:16–18, ESV

> "And this is the testimony, that God gave us eternal life, and this life is in his Son. Whoever has the Son has life; whoever does not have the Son of God does not have life."
>
> — 1 JOHN 5:11–12, ESV

> "If you confess with your mouth that Jesus is Lord and believe in your heart that God raised him from the dead, you will be saved."
>
> — ROMANS 10:9, ESV

> "If anyone is in Christ, he is a new creation; old things have passed away; behold, all things have become new."
>
> — 2 CORINTHIANS 5:17, NKJV

"Truly, truly, I say to you, whoever hears my word and believes him who sent me has eternal life. He does not come into judgment, but has passed from death to life."

— JOHN 5:24, ESV

"There is now no condemnation for those who are in Christ Jesus, because through Christ Jesus the law of the Spirit who gives life has set you free from the law of sin and death."

— ROMANS 8:1–2, NIV

"Whoever believes in the Son has eternal life; whoever does not obey the Son shall not see life, but the wrath of God remains on him."

— JOHN 3:36, ESV

"I give them eternal life, and they will never perish, and no one will snatch them out of my hand. My Father, who has given them to me, is greater than all, and no one is able to snatch them out of the Father's hand. I and the Father are one."

— JOHN 10:28–30, ESV

"For our sake he made him to be sin who knew no sin, so that in him we might become the righteousness of God."

— 2 CORINTHIANS 5:21, ESV

"We have been justified by faith, we have peace with God through our Lord Jesus Christ."

— ROMANS 5:1, ESV

"May the God of all grace, who called us to His eternal glory by Christ Jesus, after you have suffered a while, perfect, establish, strengthen and settle you."

— 1 PETER 5:10, NKJV

Prayer of faith

Jesus,

I believe Your Word that You are the Son of the living God. You loved me so much that You died in my place for my sins, then You rose again, conquering sin and death. I am sorry for my sins. I now receive Your forgiveness and Your offer of new life. I trust You to be the Lord of my life.

Amen

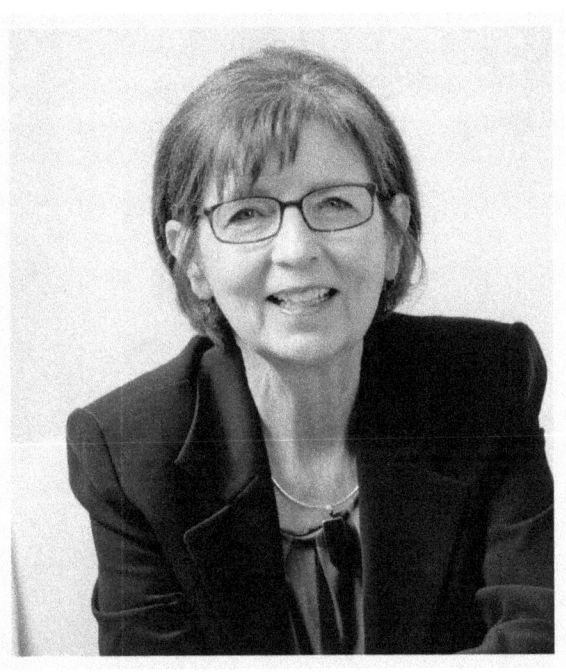

Deana Dickerson writes from her heart about her husband's ten-year cancer ordeal. Passionate about encouraging hurting people, she draws on her work in Stephen Ministry, women's mentoring programs, and her time in GriefShare and Bible study groups. Desiring to help people understand there is power for living in God's Word, this story includes those words they valued during their struggle. Retired from a healthcare career, she lives in Minneapolis and continues mentoring, writing, and traveling.

Visit the author online at salmonprairiepress.com

www.ingramcontent.com/pod-product-compliance
Lightning Source LLC
Chambersburg PA
CBHW070657100426
42735CB00039B/2175